I0767241

HOLISTIC WELLNESS: A COMPREHENSIVE GUIDE TO HEALTHY LIVING

ACHIEVE OPTIMAL HEALTH THROUGH NUTRITION, EXERCISE, SLEEP, MINDFULNESS, AND MORE

BASIL PICKARD MD

© COPYRIGHT 2024

All right reserved.

All rights reserved. No part of this publication may be reproduced, distributed, or transmitted in any form or by any means, including photocopying, recording, or other electronic or mechanical methods, without the prior written permission of the publisher, except in the case of brief quotations embodied in critical reviews and certain other noncommercial uses permitted by copyright law.

TABLE OF CONTENTS

CONCLUSION 159

INTRODUCTION

In the grand theater of life, where every day unfolds as a unique act, the central role is undeniably played by our health. Imagine the intricate machinery of your body and mind as the protagonists in a thrilling narrative, constantly adapting to the script written by our lifestyle choices. This narrative, woven with the threads of nutrition, exercise, mental well-being, and purposeful living, is what defines the epic tale of healthy living.

Healthy living isn't merely a buzzword or a fleeting trend—it is the essence that propels us towards a life of vibrancy and resilience. It's the difference between merely existing and truly thriving in the symphony of existence. Consider this: every meal you consume, every step you take, and every thought you entertain contributes to the ongoing narrative of your well-being. It's a holistic tapestry where physical vitality, mental acuity, and emotional balance converge to create a masterpiece of human experience.

In the whirlwind of our fast-paced lives, it's easy to overlook the profound impact that our choices have on our overall health. Yet, the importance of healthy living extends far beyond the superficial pursuit of an idealized body image. It is about nurturing the temple that houses our dreams, ambitions, and the very essence of who we are.

As we embark on this exploration of the blueprint for healthy living, envision it as an empowering journey—one that embraces the idea that our bodies and minds are not just vessels, but dynamic ecosystems deserving of thoughtful cultivation. Join me in uncovering the layers of this intricate tapestry, where each thread represents a conscious choice, a step towards a more vibrant, fulfilling life. The canvas is yours; let's paint a picture of health that resonates with the vitality of living fully and intentionally.

CHAPTER ONE

DEFINITION OF HEALTHY LIVING

Healthy living is a holistic approach to life that encompasses practices and choices aimed at promoting overall well-being, both physically and mentally. It involves adopting habits that contribute to the optimal functioning of the body and mind, fostering resilience, and preventing illness. Healthy living goes beyond the absence of disease and includes a balance of nutrition, regular physical activity, adequate sleep, stress management, and positive mental and emotional well-being.

A person committed to healthy living recognizes the interconnectedness of various aspects of their life, including diet, exercise, mental health, and lifestyle choices. This proactive approach emphasizes preventive measures, self-care, and conscious decision-making to enhance the quality of life and promote longevity.

In essence, healthy living is a dynamic and ongoing process that involves making informed choices to support a thriving, balanced, and sustainable lifestyle. It recognizes that health is not merely the absence of illness but a state of optimal physical, mental, and social well-being.

IMPORTANCE OF HEALTHY LIVING

The importance of healthy living cannot be overstated, as it profoundly influences various aspects of an individual's life. Here are key reasons why prioritizing healthy living is crucial:

• Physical Well-being: Healthy living promotes optimal physical health, reducing the risk of chronic diseases such as heart disease, diabetes, and obesity. Proper nutrition, regular exercise, and adequate sleep contribute to the overall well-functioning of the body.

• Mental Health: A healthy lifestyle positively impacts mental well-being. Regular exercise releases endorphins, which are known as "feel-good" hormones, contributing to improved mood and reduced stress. Adequate sleep and proper nutrition also play pivotal roles in supporting cognitive function and emotional stability.

• Energy and Vitality: Healthy living enhances energy levels and vitality, allowing individuals to engage in daily activities with vigor and enthusiasm. Nutrient-rich diets and regular exercise contribute to sustained energy throughout the day.

• Disease Prevention: Adopting a healthy lifestyle is one of the most effective ways to prevent various diseases. Eating a balanced diet, staying physically active, and avoiding harmful habits such as smoking can significantly reduce the risk of developing chronic conditions.

• Improved Immune Function: A well-balanced and nutritious diet, combined with regular exercise, supports a robust immune system. This helps the body defend against infections and illnesses, leading to fewer sick days and a quicker recovery when illnesses do occur.

• Enhanced Mental Function: Healthy living contributes to improved cognitive function, including better concentration, memory, and overall mental acuity. Proper nutrition and regular exercise support brain health and may reduce the risk of cognitive decline as individuals age.

• Stress Reduction: Engaging in healthy living practices, such as exercise, mindfulness, and adequate sleep, helps manage stress levels. Chronic stress can contribute to a range of health issues, and adopting a healthy lifestyle provides effective tools for stress management.

• Quality Sleep: Healthy living promotes good sleep hygiene, which is essential for overall health. Quality sleep is crucial for physical recovery, emotional well-being, and cognitive function.

• Longevity: Studies consistently show that individuals who adopt healthy lifestyles tend to live longer. By reducing the risk of chronic diseases and promoting overall well-being, healthy living contributes to a longer and more fulfilling life.

• Improved Quality of Life: Ultimately, healthy living enhances the overall quality of life. It allows individuals to enjoy a more active, fulfilling, and resilient existence, fostering a positive outlook and the ability to navigate life's challenges with greater ease.

In summary, the importance of healthy living lies in its multifaceted impact on physical health, mental well-being, disease prevention, and overall life satisfaction. Embracing a healthy lifestyle is an investment in one's present and future well-being.

A balanced diet plays a crucial role in maintaining and promoting optimal physical health. It provides the necessary nutrients that the body needs for various functions, growth, repair, and overall well-being. Here are key aspects of the role of a balanced diet in physical health:

• Nutrient Supply: A balanced diet ensures the intake of essential nutrients such as carbohydrates, proteins, fats, vitamins, and minerals. Each of these nutrients serves specific functions, from providing energy (carbohydrates and fats) to building and repairing tissues (proteins) and supporting various metabolic processes (vitamins and minerals).

• Energy Balance: The right balance of carbohydrates, proteins, and fats in a diet helps maintain an optimal energy balance. This balance is crucial for supporting daily activities, exercise, and overall metabolic functions. Consuming an appropriate amount of calories prevents energy imbalances that can lead to weight gain or loss.

• Weight Management: A balanced diet contributes to maintaining a healthy weight. By providing the body with the right nutrients in appropriate portions, individuals are better equipped to manage their weight, reducing the risk of obesity and related health issues, such as diabetes and cardiovascular diseases.

• Disease Prevention: A diet rich in fruits, vegetables, whole grains, lean proteins, and healthy fats is associated with a lower risk of chronic diseases. These foods provide antioxidants, fiber, and other bioactive compounds that help protect the body against conditions like heart disease, certain cancers, and diabetes.

• Bone Health: Adequate intake of calcium and vitamin D, typically found in dairy products, leafy greens, and fortified foods, supports bone health. A balanced diet helps prevent conditions like osteoporosis and ensures the maintenance of strong and healthy bones.

• Digestive Health: Fiber, present in fruits, vegetables, and whole grains, plays a crucial role in maintaining digestive health. It helps prevent constipation, supports a healthy gut microbiota, and may reduce the risk of digestive disorders.

• Immune System Support: Proper nutrition is essential for a robust immune system. Nutrients like vitamins A, C, D, and zinc, found in various foods, contribute to immune function. A balanced diet helps the body fight off infections and illnesses.

• Heart Health: Consuming a balanced diet that is low in saturated and trans fats helps promote heart health. Foods rich in omega-3 fatty acids, found in fatty fish, nuts, and seeds, can have a positive impact on cholesterol levels and reduce the risk of heart disease.

• Blood Sugar Regulation: Balanced meals with a mix of carbohydrates, proteins, and fats help regulate blood sugar levels. This is particularly important for individuals with or at risk of diabetes, as it supports glycemic control and reduces the risk of insulin resistance.

• Hydration: While not a nutrient, water is a crucial component of a balanced diet. Staying well-hydrated is essential for various bodily functions, including digestion, nutrient transport, temperature regulation, and overall cellular activity.

In summary, a balanced diet provides the necessary nutrients to support the body's physiological functions, maintain a healthy weight, prevent diseases, and promote overall well-being. It is a cornerstone of physical health and lays the foundation for a vibrant and active lifestyle.

PORTION CONTROL

Portion control is a practice of managing the amount of food you eat in a single sitting, with the aim of maintaining a healthy balance between caloric intake and energy expenditure. It is a key aspect of a healthy diet and can contribute to weight management, overall health, and prevention of various health conditions. Here are several important aspects of portion control:

• Caloric Awareness: Controlling portions helps individuals become more aware of the number of calories they consume. Understanding the energy content of different foods is essential for maintaining a healthy weight and preventing overeating.

• Weight Management: Portion control is a fundamental strategy for weight management. By moderating portion sizes, individuals can create a caloric deficit, which is essential for weight loss. Conversely, it helps prevent excess calorie intake, which can lead to weight gain.

• Balanced Nutrition: Proper portion control encourages a balanced intake of macronutrients (carbohydrates, proteins, and fats) and micronutrients (vitamins and minerals). This balance is crucial for overall health, supporting bodily functions, and preventing nutritional deficiencies.

• Preventing Overeating: Controlling portions helps prevent overeating, which can lead to discomfort, indigestion, and weight gain. It allows individuals to satisfy hunger without consuming excess calories.

• Blood Sugar Regulation: Smaller, well-controlled portions, especially when they include a mix of carbohydrates, proteins, and fats, can contribute to better blood sugar regulation. This is particularly important for individuals with diabetes or those at risk of developing insulin resistance.

• Digestive Health: Proper portion control supports good digestive health. Overeating can strain the digestive system, leading to issues such as bloating, gas, and discomfort. Smaller, well-balanced meals are easier for the digestive system to process.

• Cognitive Awareness: Portion control encourages mindful eating, where individuals pay attention to hunger and fullness cues. This mindfulness fosters a healthier relationship with food, reducing the likelihood of emotional or binge eating.

• Adaptation to Sensory Satisfaction: Over time, practicing portion control can lead to an adjustment in the perception of satisfying portions. Individuals may find that they become accustomed to smaller, more appropriate serving sizes that still provide satiety.

• Preventing Nutrient Excess: While nutrients are essential for health, excessive intake can lead to imbalances or negative health effects. Portion control helps prevent the consumption of excessive amounts of certain nutrients, such as sodium, saturated fats, or added sugars.

• Long-Term Health: Consistent portion control is associated with long-term health benefits. It contributes to maintaining a healthy weight, reducing the risk of chronic diseases (such as heart disease and diabetes), and promoting overall well-being.

Practicing portion control does not necessarily mean deprivation. It's about finding a balance that supports individual health goals and promotes a sustainable, enjoyable relationship with food. Techniques like using smaller plates, paying attention to hunger cues, and being mindful of portion sizes when dining out can help individuals incorporate effective portion control into their daily lives.

BENEFITS OF STAYING HYDRATED

Staying hydrated is crucial for maintaining overall health and well-being. Water is essential for various bodily functions, and adequate hydration offers a range of benefits. Here are some key advantages of staying hydrated:

• Regulation of Body Temperature: Water plays a vital role in thermoregulation, helping the body maintain a stable internal temperature. Adequate hydration supports the sweating process, which is the body's natural cooling mechanism.

• Improved Physical Performance: Proper hydration is essential for optimal physical performance. Dehydration can lead to fatigue, decreased endurance, and impaired strength. Athletes, in particular, benefit from staying well-hydrated to enhance their exercise performance.

• Joint Lubrication: Water is a component of synovial fluid, which lubricates joints and reduces friction between moving parts. Staying hydrated supports joint health and can alleviate discomfort associated with conditions like arthritis.

• Nutrient Transport: Water serves as a medium for the transport of nutrients throughout the body. It facilitates the absorption and distribution of essential nutrients, ensuring they reach cells and organs to support various physiological functions.

• Detoxification: Adequate hydration supports the body's natural detoxification processes by helping to flush out waste products and toxins through urine. This is essential for maintaining healthy kidneys and preventing the buildup of harmful substances.

• Cognitive Function: Dehydration can negatively impact cognitive function, including concentration, alertness, and short-term memory. Staying hydrated supports optimal brain function and may enhance mental clarity and performance.

• Digestive Health: Water is crucial for proper digestion. It helps break down food, aids in the absorption of nutrients, and prevents constipation by softening stools. Maintaining hydration is key to a healthy digestive system.

• Skin Health: Hydration plays a role in maintaining skin elasticity and preventing dryness. Dehydration can contribute to skin issues, such as flakiness and premature aging. Drinking enough water promotes a healthy complexion.

• Heart Health: Proper hydration supports cardiovascular health by maintaining blood volume and promoting optimal blood circulation. This can contribute to lower blood pressure and a reduced risk of cardiovascular diseases.

• Weight Management: Drinking water before meals can contribute to a feeling of fullness, potentially reducing calorie intake. Additionally, staying hydrated can support the body's metabolism and enhance the efficiency of metabolic processes.

• Prevention of Kidney Stones: Sufficient water intake helps dilute substances in the urine that can lead to the formation of kidney stones. Staying hydrated reduces the risk of developing these painful and potentially serious conditions.

• Mood and Energy Levels: Dehydration can contribute to feelings of fatigue and irritability. Maintaining proper hydration levels can positively influence mood and energy levels, promoting an overall sense of well-being.

It's important to note that individual hydration needs vary based on factors such as age, activity level, climate, and overall health. While there is no one-size-fits-all recommendation, a general guideline is to drink an adequate amount of water throughout the day, listening to the body's signals for thirst, and adjusting water intake based on individual circumstances.

TIPS FOR INCREASING WATER INTAKE

Increasing water intake is a simple yet effective way to enhance overall health. Here are some practical tips to help you drink more water throughout the day:

• Carry a Reusable Water Bottle: Keep a reusable water bottle with you wherever you go. Having it readily available makes it easier to sip water consistently throughout the day.

• Set Reminders: Use phone alarms or reminders to prompt you to drink water at regular intervals. This can be especially helpful if you have a busy schedule.

• Flavor Your Water: If plain water doesn't appeal to you, try infusing it with natural flavors. Add slices of lemon, cucumber, mint, or berries to enhance the taste without adding calories or sugar.

• Create a Water Schedule: Establish specific times during the day for drinking water. For example, have a glass of water when you wake up, before meals, and before bedtime.

• Use an App: Several mobile apps are designed to help you track and increase your water intake. These apps often send reminders and provide a visual representation of your daily progress.

• Try Herbal Tea: Herbal teas, whether hot or cold, can contribute to your overall fluid intake. Choose caffeine-free options for the best hydration benefits.

• Eat Water-Rich Foods: Consume foods with high water content, such as watermelon, cucumber, celery, oranges, and strawberries. These foods not only hydrate but also provide additional nutrients.

• Pair Water with Activities: Link drinking water with specific activities, such as taking a sip after answering emails or during breaks. This helps create a routine and makes hydration a habit.

• Invest in a Fun Water Pitcher: If you prefer drinking from a pitcher, choose one with a design or feature that makes the process enjoyable. This can be a visual reminder to drink more.

• Track Your Progress: Keep a log or use a hydration tracking app to monitor your daily water intake. Seeing your progress can be motivating and help you reach your hydration goals.

• Make it a Ritual: Create a small ritual around drinking water, such as using a favorite glass or taking a moment to enjoy a refreshing sip. This can make the experience more enjoyable.

• Alternate with Other Beverages: If you enjoy other beverages like herbal teas or diluted fruit juices, alternate them with water to increase overall fluid intake while keeping variety in your drinks.

Remember that individual water needs vary, and factors like age, climate, and physical activity levels influence how much water you should drink. Pay attention to your body's signals, and aim to maintain a balance that suits your lifestyle and health goals.

TYPES OF EXERCISE FOR PHYSICAL HEALTH

Engaging in a variety of exercises is key to promoting overall physical health. Different types of exercise offer various benefits and contribute to overall fitness. Here are several types of exercises for physical health:

Aerobic or Cardiovascular Exercises:

• Examples: Running, walking, cycling, swimming, dancing.

• Benefits: Improves cardiovascular health, enhances endurance, burns calories, and supports weight management.

Strength Training:

• Examples: Weight lifting, resistance band exercises, bodyweight exercises (e.g., squats, push-ups).

• Benefits: Builds muscle strength, increases metabolism, supports joint health, and enhances overall functional fitness.

• Examples: Yoga, Pilates, static stretching, dynamic stretching.

• Benefits: Improves flexibility, enhances joint range of motion, reduces muscle tension, and may prevent injuries.

• Examples: Tai Chi, balance exercises on one leg, stability ball exercises.

• Benefits: Enhances balance and coordination, strengthens stabilizing muscles, reduces the risk of falls, and supports functional movement.

• Examples: Short bursts of intense exercise followed by periods of rest or lower-intensity activity.

• Benefits: Improves cardiovascular fitness, burns calories efficiently, and can be time-effective.

• Examples: Swimming, cycling, elliptical training.

• Benefits: Provides cardiovascular benefits with reduced impact on joints, making it suitable for individuals with joint concerns.

CrossFit or Functional Training:

• Examples: Varied exercises combining elements of strength training, cardiovascular exercise, and flexibility.

• Benefits: Enhances overall fitness, improves strength, endurance, and agility, and mimics real-life movements.

Interval Training:

• Examples: Alternating between short bursts of high-intensity exercise and periods of lower-intensity or rest.

• Benefits: Boosts cardiovascular fitness, burns calories, and can be adaptable to various forms of exercise.

Circuit Training:

• Examples: Performing a series of exercises in sequence with minimal rest between each.

• Benefits: Combines strength and cardiovascular elements, enhances overall fitness, and can be time-efficient.

Group Exercise Classes:

• Examples: Spinning classes, aerobics, Zumba, group fitness classes.

• Benefits: Provides social interaction, motivation, and structured workouts led by instructors.

Outdoor Activities:

• Examples: Hiking, trail running, kayaking, biking.

• Benefits: Combines exercise with exposure to nature, offering mental health benefits along with physical activity.

Mind-Body Exercises:

• Examples: Yoga, Tai Chi, Qi Gong.

• Benefits: Integrates physical movement with mindfulness, promoting relaxation, flexibility, and stress reduction.

Remember, it's important to incorporate a mix of these exercises into your routine to target various aspects of physical health, including cardiovascular fitness, strength, flexibility, and overall well-being. Consult with a healthcare professional or fitness expert before starting a new exercise program, especially if you have pre-existing health conditions or concerns.

REGULAR PHYSICAL ACTIVITY

Regular physical activity is a cornerstone of a healthy lifestyle and offers a multitude of benefits for both physical and mental well-being. Here are key aspects and advantages of incorporating regular physical activity into your routine:

• Cardiovascular Health: Regular aerobic exercises such as brisk walking, running, or cycling help improve cardiovascular health. They strengthen the heart, enhance circulation, and lower the risk of heart diseases.

• Weight Management: Physical activity plays a crucial role in weight management by burning calories and increasing metabolism. Combining regular exercise with a balanced diet can contribute to maintaining a healthy weight.

• Muscle Strength and Endurance: Strength training exercises, including weightlifting and resistance training, promote the development of muscle strength and endurance. This contributes to improved overall functional fitness.

• Bone Health: Weight-bearing exercises like walking, jogging, and resistance training are beneficial for bone health. They help maintain bone density and reduce the risk of osteoporosis.

• Improved Flexibility and Range of Motion: Activities such as yoga and stretching exercises enhance flexibility and joint range of motion. This can improve posture, reduce the risk of injuries, and contribute to overall mobility.

• Enhanced Mood and Mental Well-being: Physical activity stimulates the release of endorphins, neurotransmitters that contribute to feelings of happiness and reduced stress. Regular exercise is associated with improved mood, reduced anxiety, and better mental well-being.

• Better Sleep Quality: Engaging in regular physical activity can promote better sleep patterns and overall sleep quality. It helps regulate circadian rhythms and can be beneficial for individuals with sleep disorders.

• Reduced Risk of Chronic Diseases: Regular physical activity is linked to a lower risk of chronic diseases such as type 2 diabetes, certain cancers, and metabolic syndrome. It also helps manage existing health conditions.

• Improved Immune Function: Moderate and regular exercise has been shown to enhance immune function, reducing the risk of infections and promoting overall immune system health.

• Increased Energy Levels: Regular physical activity boosts energy levels by improving circulation and increasing oxygen flow to tissues. This results in increased stamina and reduced feelings of fatigue.

• Enhanced Cognitive Function: Exercise is associated with improved cognitive function, including better memory, attention, and processing speed. It may also contribute to a reduced risk of cognitive decline as individuals age.

• Social Interaction: Participating in group activities, sports, or fitness classes provides opportunities for social interaction. Building connections with others through physical activity can enhance mental well-being and motivation.

• Stress Management: Exercise serves as a powerful stress management tool. Physical activity helps reduce levels of stress hormones and provides a healthy outlet for coping with life's challenges.

• Longevity: Regular physical activity is linked to increased life expectancy. Adopting an active lifestyle contributes to a longer and healthier life.

To reap the full benefits of regular physical activity, it's important to choose activities that you enjoy and that align with your fitness level and goals. Aim for a mix of aerobic, strength training, and flexibility exercises throughout the week, and consider consulting with a healthcare professional or fitness expert for personalized guidance.

STRENGTH TRAINING AND FLEXIBILITY

Strength training and flexibility exercises are two essential components of a well-rounded fitness routine, each offering unique benefits for overall physical health and fitness. Let's explore the importance of each:

• Muscle Development: Strength training involves lifting weights or using resistance to challenge muscles. This leads to the development and growth of muscle tissues, improving overall strength and tone.

• Metabolic Boost: Building muscle contributes to an increase in resting metabolic rate. This means that, even at rest, individuals with more muscle mass burn more calories, which can be beneficial for weight management.

• Bone Health: Resistance training is beneficial for bone health. It helps increase bone density and can reduce the risk of osteoporosis and fractures, especially in older adults.

• Improved Joint Function: Strengthening the muscles around joints provides better support, reducing the risk of injuries and promoting joint stability. This is particularly important for individuals with joint issues or arthritis.

• Enhanced Functional Fitness: Strength training exercises mimic real-life movements, improving functional fitness. This is crucial for activities like lifting, carrying, and maintaining balance in daily life.

• Fatigue Resistance: Regular strength training can enhance endurance and reduce the perception of fatigue during various activities, contributing to improved overall fitness.

• Weight Management: Building muscle contributes to a leaner body composition, which can be beneficial for weight management. It also helps shape and define the physique.

• Improved Posture: Strengthening the muscles of the core, back, and shoulders promotes better posture. This can alleviate common issues associated with poor posture, such as back pain.

Flexibility:

• Increased Range of Motion: Flexibility exercises, including stretching and yoga, improve the range of motion in joints. This is crucial for maintaining overall mobility and preventing stiffness.

• Reduced Muscle Tension: Stretching helps release muscle tension, reducing feelings of tightness and discomfort. It can alleviate stiffness, especially after periods of inactivity.

• Injury Prevention: Flexible muscles and joints are less prone to injury. Incorporating flexibility exercises into a routine helps improve muscle and joint resilience, reducing the risk of strains and sprains.

• Enhanced Circulation: Stretching improves blood flow to muscles, enhancing circulation. This can contribute to better nutrient delivery to tissues and improved recovery after exercise.

• Stress Reduction: Engaging in flexibility exercises often incorporates relaxation techniques, promoting mental well-being and stress reduction. Practices like yoga, in particular, focus on the mind-body connection.

• Improved Balance and Coordination: Enhanced flexibility contributes to better balance and coordination. This is beneficial for overall stability and can reduce the risk of falls, especially in older adults.

• Better Posture: Stretching exercises, particularly those targeting muscles involved in posture, can contribute to improved alignment and reduced strain on the spine.

• Joint Health: Maintaining flexibility is crucial for joint health. It helps prevent stiffness and supports the lubrication of joints, promoting overall joint function.

Incorporating both strength training and flexibility exercises into your fitness routine provides a comprehensive approach to physical health. Whether through weightlifting, resistance training, yoga, or dynamic stretching, combining these elements contributes to improved strength, mobility, and overall well-being. Always start with proper warm-up exercises before engaging in strength or flexibility training, and consider consulting with a fitness professional for personalized guidance, especially if you are new to these activities.

CHAPTER TWO

IMPORTANCE OF SLEEP

Sleep is a fundamental aspect of overall health and well-being, playing a crucial role in various physiological and cognitive functions. Here are some key reasons highlighting the importance of sleep:

Physical Health:

• Recovery and Repair: Sleep is a period during which the body undergoes repair and recovery processes. Tissues are repaired, muscles are rebuilt, and various cells are regenerated.

• Immune System Support: Adequate sleep is essential for a robust immune system. During sleep, the body produces cytokines and antibodies that help fight off infections and illnesses.

• Hormone Regulation: Sleep plays a vital role in regulating hormones, including those that control stress, growth, appetite, and metabolism. Disruptions in sleep can affect hormone balance, potentially leading to various health issues.

• Weight Management: Lack of sleep has been linked to disruptions in hunger hormones, such as ghrelin and leptin. This can contribute to increased appetite and a higher likelihood of weight gain.

• Heart Health: Chronic sleep deprivation is associated with an increased risk of cardiovascular diseases, including hypertension, heart attack, and stroke.

• Blood Sugar Regulation: Adequate sleep is crucial for maintaining proper glucose metabolism. Sleep deprivation can lead to insulin resistance and an increased risk of type 2 diabetes.

Mental Health:

• Cognitive Function: Sleep is essential for cognitive processes such as memory consolidation, learning, and problem-solving. A good night's sleep enhances attention, creativity, and overall cognitive performance.

• Emotional Well-being: Lack of sleep is linked to mood disturbances, including irritability, anxiety, and feelings of stress. Quality sleep contributes to emotional resilience and a more positive outlook.

• Stress Reduction: Sleep plays a key role in stress management. Adequate sleep helps regulate the body's stress response system, reducing the impact of stressors on mental and emotional well-being.

• Mental Health Disorders: Chronic sleep deprivation is associated with an increased risk of developing mental health disorders such as depression and anxiety. Conversely, addressing sleep issues can be part of the treatment for these conditions.

• Regulation of Neurotransmitters: Sleep is essential for the regulation of neurotransmitters, including serotonin and dopamine. Proper neurotransmitter balance is crucial for mood stability and mental health.

Performance and Daily Functioning:

• Alertness and Concentration: Quality sleep enhances alertness, attention, and concentration. This is vital for optimal performance in daily activities, work, and academic pursuits.

• Motor Skills and Coordination: Adequate sleep is necessary for maintaining motor skills and coordination. Lack of sleep can impair reaction times and increase the risk of accidents.

- Decision-Making: Sleep influences higher-order cognitive functions, including decision-making and judgment. Well-rested individuals tend to make better decisions than those who are sleep-deprived.

- Productivity: Good sleep hygiene positively impacts productivity. Well-rested individuals are generally more efficient, focused, and capable of completing tasks in a timely manner.

In summary, sleep is a critical component of a healthy lifestyle, influencing both physical and mental well-being. Prioritizing good sleep hygiene and ensuring an adequate amount of sleep each night is essential for overall health, resilience, and optimal daily functioning.

ESTABLISHING A SLEEP ROUTINE

Establishing a consistent sleep routine, also known as a bedtime routine, can be instrumental in improving sleep quality and promoting overall well-being. Here are some steps you can take to create an effective sleep routine:

• Set a Consistent Sleep Schedule: Go to bed and wake up at the same time every day, even on weekends. Consistency helps regulate your body's internal clock, making it easier to fall asleep and wake up naturally.

• Create a Relaxing Bedtime Ritual: Develop a calming routine before bedtime to signal to your body that it's time to wind down. This can include activities such as reading a book, taking a warm bath, practicing relaxation exercises, or gentle stretching.

• Establish a Comfortable Sleep Environment: Make your bedroom conducive to sleep. Ensure the room is dark, quiet, and cool. Invest in a comfortable mattress and pillows. Consider using blackout curtains, earplugs, or a white noise machine to minimize disruptions.

• Limit Exposure to Screens Before Bed: Avoid electronic devices such as smartphones, tablets, and computers at least an hour before bedtime. The blue light emitted from screens can interfere with the production of the sleep-inducing hormone melatonin.

• Mind Your Diet: Avoid heavy meals, caffeine, and nicotine close to bedtime. These substances can disrupt sleep patterns and make it harder to fall asleep.

• Stay Active During the Day: Engage in regular physical activity, but try to finish your workout at least a few hours before bedtime. Exercise promotes better sleep, but vigorous activity too close to bedtime can be stimulating.

• Manage Stress: Practice stress-reducing techniques such as meditation, deep breathing, or progressive muscle relaxation. Managing stress can contribute to a more relaxed state before bedtime.

• Limit Naps: If you need to nap during the day, keep it short (20-30 minutes) and avoid napping too close to bedtime, as it may interfere with nighttime sleep.

• Use Your Bed for Sleep: Reserve your bed for sleep and intimate activities only. Avoid using it for work or other stimulating activities to strengthen the association between your bed and sleep.

• Create a Pre-Sleep Routine: Wind down gradually before bedtime. Dim the lights, engage in calming activities, and avoid stimulating conversations or activities.

• Limit Liquid Intake Before Bed: Minimize the consumption of liquids close to bedtime to reduce the likelihood of waking up for bathroom trips during the night.

• Seek Natural Light Exposure: Get exposure to natural light during the day, especially in the morning. Natural light helps regulate your body's circadian rhythm, promoting wakefulness during the day and better sleep at night.

• Limit Clock Watching: Avoid constantly checking the clock during the night. This can create anxiety and make it harder to fall back asleep if you wake up.

• Address Sleep Disorders: If you consistently struggle with sleep, consider consulting a healthcare professional. Conditions such as insomnia or sleep apnea may require specialized treatment.

By consistently following a sleep routine and incorporating these practices, you can train your body to associate specific behaviors with sleep and create a conducive environment for restful nights. It may take some time for your body to adjust, so be patient and stay committed to your routine.

STRESSORS IDENTIFICATION

Identifying stressors is a crucial step in managing and mitigating stress. Understanding the sources of stress in your life allows you to develop effective coping strategies. Here are steps to help you identify and manage stressors:

• Self-Reflection: Take time for self-reflection to identify situations, events, or circumstances that trigger stress. Consider recent experiences where you felt overwhelmed or anxious.

• Keep a Stress Journal: Maintain a stress journal to record daily stressors. Note the events, your emotional responses, and how you coped. Over time, patterns may emerge, helping you identify recurring stressors.

• Categorize Stressors: Group stressors into categories such as work, relationships, financial, health, and personal. This helps you recognize broader patterns and prioritize areas for intervention.

• Physical Symptoms: Pay attention to physical signs of stress, such as headaches, muscle tension, or digestive issues. These symptoms can provide clues about the sources of stress in your life.

• Emotional Responses: Monitor your emotional responses to different situations. Identify instances where you feel consistently anxious, irritable, or overwhelmed. Emotional reactions can be indicators of underlying stressors.

• Life Changes: Major life changes, both positive and negative, can be significant stressors. Events like job changes, moving, relationship transitions, or loss can impact your stress levels.

• Time Management: Evaluate your schedule and workload. Identify tasks or commitments that consistently create time pressure and stress. Consider ways to prioritize and manage your time more effectively.

• Relationships: Assess your relationships, both personal and professional. Identify dynamics that contribute to stress. This may include conflicts, communication challenges, or unrealistic expectations.

• Financial Pressures: Financial concerns can be a significant stressor. Identify specific financial challenges and explore strategies for budgeting, saving, or seeking financial advice.

• Environmental Factors: Evaluate your physical environment. Noisy or cluttered spaces, lack of privacy, or uncomfortable surroundings can contribute to stress. Identify changes that could improve your environment.

• Workplace Stressors: Examine your work environment for stressors. High workload, unrealistic expectations, lack of control, or conflict with colleagues can contribute to workplace stress.

• Health Factors: Consider how health-related issues impact your stress levels. Chronic health conditions, lack of exercise, poor nutrition, or inadequate sleep can contribute to overall stress.

• Unrealistic Expectations: Reflect on whether you set unrealistic expectations for yourself or others. Unrealistic goals or perfectionism can be sources of stress.

• Social Media and Information Overload: Assess the role of social media and information overload in your life. Constant exposure to news, social comparison, or excessive screen time can contribute to stress.

• Lack of Self-Care: Identify areas where you may be neglecting self-care. Lack of relaxation, leisure, and activities you enjoy can contribute to stress.

• Consult Others: Seek input from friends, family, or colleagues. Sometimes, others can provide valuable insights into stressors that you may not have fully recognized.

• Professional Help: If stressors seem overwhelming or persist, consider seeking the assistance of a mental health professional. They can provide guidance and support in coping with and managing stress.

By systematically examining various aspects of your life and paying attention to physical, emotional, and environmental cues, you can identify stressors and develop targeted strategies to address them. It's important to recognize that stress management is an ongoing process, and regularly reassessing your stressors is essential for maintaining well-being.

Relaxation techniques are effective ways to manage stress, promote a sense of calm, and enhance overall well-being. Incorporating these practices into your routine can help you relax both your mind and body. Here are some relaxation techniques to consider:

1. Deep Breathing:

• Technique: Sit or lie down comfortably. Inhale slowly through your nose, allowing your chest and abdomen to rise. Exhale slowly through your mouth, letting the breath out completely.

• Purpose: Deep breathing triggers the body's relaxation response, reducing stress and promoting a sense of calm.

2. Progressive Muscle Relaxation (PMR):

• Technique: Systematically tense and then relax different muscle groups. Start with your toes and work your way up to your head.

• Purpose: PMR helps release physical tension, promoting relaxation throughout the body.

3. Guided Imagery:

- Technique: Close your eyes and imagine a peaceful scene or scenario. Use all your senses to create a vivid mental image.

- Purpose: Guided imagery can shift your focus away from stressors and create a calming mental space.

4. Mindfulness Meditation:

- Technique: Focus your attention on your breath or a specific object. Allow thoughts to come and go without judgment, bringing your attention back to the present moment.

- Purpose: Mindfulness meditation cultivates awareness, reduces stress, and enhances mental clarity.

5. Autogenic Training:

- Technique: Repeat a series of self-statements about warmth and heaviness in different parts of your body.

- Purpose: Autogenic training helps induce a state of physical relaxation and mental calmness.

6. Yoga:

• Technique: Engage in yoga poses, combining movement, breath, and mindfulness. Focus on the mind-body connection.

• Purpose: Yoga promotes flexibility, relaxation, and stress reduction.

7. Tai Chi:

• Technique: Perform slow, deliberate movements while focusing on your breath. Tai Chi is often described as "meditation in motion."

• Purpose: Tai Chi helps improve balance, reduce tension, and promote a sense of peace.

8. Aromatherapy:

• Technique: Use essential oils, such as lavender or chamomile, through diffusion or massage. Inhale the calming scents.

• Purpose: Aromatherapy can have a soothing effect on the mind and body.

9. Listening to Calming Music:

• Technique: Choose music with a slow tempo and calming melodies. Listen mindfully, paying attention to the music.

• Purpose: Music has the power to influence mood and induce relaxation.

10. Warm Baths:

• Technique: Take a warm bath with Epsom salts or calming essential oils.

• Purpose: Warm baths help relax tense muscles and create a soothing environment.

11. Journaling:

• Technique: Write down your thoughts, feelings, and experiences. Use a journal as an emotional outlet.

• Purpose: Journaling can help process emotions and gain perspective, promoting relaxation.

12. Breath Focus in Nature:

• Technique: Find a quiet outdoor spot. Sit or stand comfortably, and focus on your breath while observing the sights and sounds of nature.

• Purpose: Connecting with nature can have a calming effect on the mind.

13. Humor and Laughter:

• Technique: Watch a funny movie, read a humorous book, or spend time with people who make you laugh.

• Purpose: Laughter releases endorphins, the body's natural feel-good chemicals, promoting relaxation.

14. Sensory Relaxation:

• Technique: Engage your senses in a calming way, such as feeling a soft fabric, tasting a soothing tea, or enjoying a gentle massage.

• Purpose: Sensory experiences can shift your focus and induce relaxation.

15. Breath Counting:

• Technique: Inhale deeply, count to four, and exhale completely. Gradually increase the count as you become more comfortable.

• Purpose: Breath counting helps focus the mind and regulate breathing for relaxation.

Experiment with different relaxation techniques to find what works best for you. Incorporate these practices into your daily routine or use them as needed during stressful moments to foster a sense of calm and balance.

MINDFULNESS AND MEDITATION

Mindfulness and meditation are practices that involve cultivating awareness, presence, and a focused state of mind. They have been shown to have numerous mental, emotional, and physical health benefits. Here's an overview of mindfulness and meditation:

Mindfulness:

- Definition: Mindfulness is the practice of bringing one's attention to the present moment with an attitude of openness, curiosity, and acceptance.

Basic Principles:

- Observation: Paying attention to thoughts, feelings, and sensations without judgment.

- Non-Attachment: Allowing experiences to come and go without becoming overly attached or reactive.

Key Elements:

- Breath Awareness: Focusing on the breath as it goes in and out.

- Body Scan: Bringing attention to different parts of the body.

- Observing Thoughts: Noticing thoughts without becoming entangled in them.

- Mindful Walking or Eating: Engaging in activities with full attention.

Benefits:

• Stress Reduction: Mindfulness helps manage stress by cultivating a non-reactive awareness of challenging situations.

• Improved Focus: Regular practice enhances attention and concentration.

• Emotional Regulation: Mindfulness fosters a balanced and non-reactive approach to emotions.

• Enhanced Well-being: It contributes to an overall sense of well-being and improved quality of life.

Meditation:

• Definition: Meditation is a intentional practice where an individual uses a technique – such as mindfulness, focused attention, or loving-kindness – to train attention and awareness, and achieve a mentally clear and emotionally calm state.

Types of Meditation:

• Mindfulness Meditation: Focusing on the present moment and observing thoughts and sensations.

• Loving-Kindness Meditation (Metta): Cultivating feelings of love and compassion toward oneself and others.

• Transcendental Meditation (TM): Using a mantra to achieve a state of restful alertness.

• Guided Meditation: Following the guidance of a teacher or recording through a specific visualization or mindfulness exercise.

Basic Principles:

• Focus: Concentrating attention on a chosen point, such as the breath, a mantra, or an object.

• Non-Judgmental Awareness: Observing thoughts without judgment and gently bringing the mind back when it wanders.

Benefits:

• Stress Reduction: Meditation helps activate the relaxation response, reducing the production of stress hormones.

• Improved Concentration: Regular practice enhances the ability to sustain attention.

• Emotional Well-being: Meditation contributes to emotional regulation and a more positive outlook.

• Mind-Body Connection: It promotes a deeper connection between the mind and body.

Mindfulness Meditation:

• Integration of Mindfulness and Meditation: Mindfulness meditation often combines elements of both mindfulness and meditation practices. It involves cultivating awareness while using a specific meditation technique.

• Guided Mindfulness Meditation: Some mindfulness meditations are guided, providing verbal instructions to direct attention and promote relaxation.

• Mindfulness-Based Stress Reduction (MBSR): MBSR is a structured program that integrates mindfulness meditation and yoga to reduce stress and enhance well-being.

• Start Small: Begin with short sessions, gradually increasing the duration as you become more comfortable.

• Consistency is Key: Regular practice, even for a few minutes each day, is more beneficial than sporadic, longer sessions.

• Find a Quiet Space: Choose a quiet and comfortable space where you can practice without distractions.

• Use Resources: Consider using guided meditations or mindfulness apps to support your practice.

• Be Patient: Mindfulness and meditation are skills that develop over time. Be patient with yourself and your progress.

• Explore Different Approaches: Try different types of meditation to find what resonates with you. Whether it's mindfulness, loving-kindness, or another technique, there are various approaches to explore.

Both mindfulness and meditation offer valuable tools for managing stress, promoting mental clarity, and enhancing overall well-being. Incorporating these practices into your daily life can lead to a greater sense of calm, increased self-awareness, and improved resilience in the face of life's challenges.

OPEN COMMUNICATION

Open communication is a key component of healthy relationships, whether in personal, professional, or social contexts. It involves expressing thoughts, feelings, and ideas in a transparent and honest manner. Here are essential elements and tips for fostering open communication:

Elements of Open Communication:

Honesty:

• Definition: Truthfulness and sincerity in expressing thoughts and feelings.

• Importance: Honesty builds trust and creates a foundation for open communication.

Clarity:

• Definition: Clearly expressing ideas to avoid misunderstandings.

• Importance: Clarity promotes effective communication and reduces the likelihood of misinterpretation.

Active Listening:

• Definition: Fully concentrating, understanding, responding, and remembering what the other person is saying.

• Importance: Active listening fosters understanding and demonstrates respect for the speaker's perspective.

Respect:

• Definition: Valuing the opinions and feelings of others, even if they differ from your own.

• Importance: Respectful communication encourages open dialogue and cooperation.

Empathy:

• Definition: Understanding and sharing the feelings of another person.

• Importance: Empathy creates a connection, fostering a supportive and compassionate communication environment.

Feedback:

• Definition: Providing constructive feedback and being open to receiving it.

• Importance: Constructive feedback contributes to personal and professional growth and enhances communication effectiveness.

Non-Verbal Communication:

• Definition: Body language, facial expressions, and gestures that convey messages.

• Importance: Non-verbal cues can complement or contradict verbal communication, impacting overall understanding.

Open-Mindedness:

• Definition: Being receptive to different perspectives and ideas.

• Importance: Open-mindedness encourages diverse thinking and fosters creativity in problem-solving.

Tips for Fostering Open Communication:

• Create a Safe Environment: Encourage an atmosphere where individuals feel safe expressing themselves without fear of judgment or reprisal.

• Be Clear and Concise: Clearly articulate your thoughts to minimize misunderstandings. Use straightforward language and avoid unnecessary complexity.

• Practice Active Listening: Give your full attention to the speaker, ask clarifying questions, and paraphrase to ensure you've understood correctly.

• Express Yourself Honestly: Share your thoughts and feelings openly, providing others with insight into your perspective.

• Use "I" Statements: Frame statements in terms of your feelings and experiences to avoid sounding accusatory. For example, say "I feel" rather than "You always."

• Encourage Feedback: Invite others to share their thoughts and encourage constructive feedback. Create an environment where feedback is seen as an opportunity for growth.

• Avoid Assumptions: Clarify and verify information rather than making assumptions. Misunderstandings often arise from assumptions.

• Manage Emotions: Acknowledge and manage your emotions during communication. If emotions escalate, consider taking a break before continuing the conversation.

• Be Open to Change: Embrace new ideas and be willing to adjust your perspective based on the information shared during the communication process.

• Seek Common Ground: Identify areas of agreement and shared values to build understanding and foster cooperation.

• Encourage Diverse Perspectives: Appreciate and seek out diverse viewpoints. Embrace the richness that different perspectives bring to the conversation.

• Practice Patience: Allow others the time they need to express themselves. Avoid interrupting or rushing the conversation.

• Use Positive Body Language: Pay attention to your body language, ensuring it aligns with your verbal communication. Maintain eye contact and use open and inviting gestures.

• Follow Up: After a conversation, follow up to ensure clarity and address any lingering questions or concerns.

Open communication is a continuous process that requires effort and commitment from all parties involved. By fostering a culture of openness, trust, and respect, individuals and groups can build stronger, healthier relationships and work collaboratively towards shared goals.

HEALTHY RELATIONSHIPS

Healthy relationships are built on a foundation of mutual respect, trust, communication, and support. Whether in personal, romantic, familial, or professional contexts, the principles of a healthy relationship remain consistent. Here are key elements and tips for cultivating and maintaining healthy relationships:

Key Elements of Healthy Relationships:

• Open and Honest Communication: Regularly share thoughts, feelings, and concerns with transparency. Foster an environment where both parties feel comfortable expressing themselves.

• Mutual Respect: Value each other's opinions, boundaries, and autonomy. Treat each other with kindness and consideration.

• Reliability and Accountability: Build trust through consistent and reliable behavior. Hold yourself and others accountable for commitments.

• Understanding and Empathy: Be attuned to each other's emotions and perspectives. Show empathy and compassion during challenging times.

• Respecting Boundaries: Establish and respect personal and relational boundaries. Recognize and communicate your own boundaries while acknowledging and honoring those of others.

• Equal Partnership: Strive for equality in decision-making, responsibilities, and power dynamics. Healthy relationships are partnerships where both individuals contribute and have a voice.

• Emotional Support: Offer emotional support during both good and challenging times. Be each other's cheerleader and provide encouragement.

• Spending Quality Time Together: Dedicate time to nurture the relationship. Engage in activities that bring joy and strengthen the connection.

• Supporting Individual Growth: Encourage personal growth and development. Healthy relationships allow individuals to pursue their goals and aspirations.

• Effective Conflict Resolution: Address conflicts with respect and a willingness to understand each other's perspectives. Seek solutions collaboratively.

• Expressing Appreciation: Regularly express gratitude and appreciation for each other's contributions and qualities.

• Alignment of Values: Build relationships with individuals who share core values and life goals. Common values contribute to long-term compatibility.

Tips for Cultivating Healthy Relationships:

• Effective Communication: Practice active listening, avoid assumptions, and use "I" statements to express your feelings and needs.

• Regular Check-Ins: Set aside time for regular check-ins to discuss the state of the relationship, address concerns, and share positive experiences.

• Quality Time: Prioritize spending quality time together. This can involve shared activities, meaningful conversations, or simply enjoying each other's company.

• Encourage Independence: Foster each other's individuality. Encourage personal pursuits, interests, and friendships outside the relationship.

• Apologize and Forgive: Be willing to apologize when necessary and forgive. Holding onto grudges can erode the foundation of a healthy relationship.

• Celebrate Achievements: Celebrate each other's successes and milestones. Acknowledge and support each other's achievements.

• Adaptability: Be adaptable to life changes and challenges. Flexibility in navigating obstacles contributes to the resilience of the relationship.

• Seek Professional Help: If challenges arise that seem insurmountable, consider seeking the guidance of a relationship counselor or therapist.

• Maintain Independence: While being part of a relationship, maintain a sense of self. Nurture your own interests, friendships, and personal growth.

• Healthy Boundaries: Clearly communicate and respect boundaries. This ensures that both individuals feel secure and understood in the relationship.

• Shared Goals: Discuss and align on shared goals, both short-term and long-term. This helps create a sense of direction and purpose.

• Mindful Conflict Resolution: Approach conflicts with a focus on understanding, resolution, and growth. Avoid blame and criticism, and instead, work together to find solutions.

• Continuous Growth: Embrace the idea that relationships are dynamic and require ongoing effort. Commit to continuous personal and relational growth.

Remember that healthy relationships are a continuous process of nurturing, understanding, and adapting. They thrive on mutual effort, respect, and a shared commitment to building a supportive and fulfilling connection.

SEEKING SUPPORT WHEN NEEDED

Seeking support when needed is a crucial aspect of maintaining mental, emotional, and physical well-being. Whether facing personal challenges, dealing with stress, or navigating significant life changes, reaching out for support can provide valuable assistance and perspective. Here are some considerations and tips for seeking support:

1. Recognizing the Need for Support:

• Self-Reflection: Pay attention to your thoughts, emotions, and overall well-being. If you notice persistent feelings of overwhelm, sadness, anxiety, or other concerns, it may be a sign that you could benefit from support.

2. Types of Support:

• Friends and Family: Trusted friends and family members can offer emotional support, understanding, and a listening ear.

• Professional Support: Therapists, counselors, psychologists, or psychiatrists can provide specialized assistance for mental health concerns.

• Support Groups: Connecting with others who share similar experiences can provide a sense of community and understanding.

• Mentors or Advisors: Seeking guidance from mentors or advisors can be beneficial for professional or personal development.

3. Overcoming Stigma:

• Normalize Seeking Help: Understand that seeking support is a sign of strength, not weakness. Everyone faces challenges, and reaching out for assistance is a positive step toward growth and well-being.

4. Choosing the Right Support System:

• Identify Trusted Individuals: Choose individuals who are supportive, non-judgmental, and have your best interests at heart.

5. Communication:

• Express Your Needs Clearly: Clearly communicate your needs and the type of support you are seeking. Be open and honest about your feelings and concerns.

6. Professional Support:

• Therapy or Counseling: If facing mental health challenges, consider reaching out to a mental health professional for specialized support and guidance.

7. Peer Support:

• Support Groups or Communities: Connect with people who have faced similar challenges. Shared experiences can foster understanding and empathy.

8. Online Resources:

• Helplines and Online Platforms: Utilize helplines, online forums, or mental health apps that provide information, resources, and a platform to connect with others.

9. Set Realistic Expectations:

• Understand the Limitations: Recognize that not everyone may be equipped to provide the support you need. It's okay to seek professional assistance when necessary.

10. Regular Check-Ins:

• Monitor Your Well-Being: Regularly check in with yourself to assess your mental and emotional well-being. If you notice persistent challenges, consider seeking support proactively.

11. Encourage Others to Seek Help:

• Normalize Support in Your Community: Foster a culture of openness and support by encouraging others to seek help when needed. Share your own experiences if you feel comfortable.

12. Be Patient with Yourself:

• Seeking Support Takes Time: Understand that finding the right support system may take time. Be patient with the process and give yourself credit for taking steps toward well-being.

13. Confidentiality:

• Ensure Privacy: If privacy is a concern, clarify with the support system that you expect confidentiality and discuss any boundaries around sharing information.

14. Explore Different Options:

• Try Different Approaches: If one form of support doesn't feel effective, be open to exploring different options until you find what works best for you.

Remember that seeking support is a proactive and positive step toward taking care of yourself. It demonstrates self-awareness and a commitment to your well-being. Whether it's through informal conversations with friends or family, professional therapy, or support groups, finding the right support system can contribute significantly to navigating life's challenges.

CONTINUOUS LEARNING

Continuous learning is a lifelong process of acquiring new knowledge, skills, and experiences. It goes beyond formal education and involves a commitment to personal and professional development throughout one's life. Here are key aspects and tips for embracing continuous learning:

Key Aspects of Continuous Learning:

• Adaptability: Continuous learning fosters adaptability by helping individuals stay relevant in a rapidly changing world. It enables them to embrace new technologies, methodologies, and ideas.

• Skill Development: Individuals can enhance existing skills and acquire new ones, whether they are related to their current profession or personal interests.

• Professional Growth: Continuous learning contributes to professional growth and career advancement. It can lead to increased job satisfaction, expanded responsibilities, and access to new opportunities.

• Intellectual Curiosity: A commitment to continuous learning is fueled by intellectual curiosity—a desire to explore, understand, and stay informed about various subjects.

• Problem-Solving: Continuous learners develop strong problem-solving skills, as they are accustomed to seeking information, analyzing situations, and finding innovative solutions.

• Versatility: Learning continuously makes individuals versatile, capable of adapting to different roles and responsibilities, which is valuable in dynamic work environments.

• Personal Enrichment: Beyond professional development, continuous learning enriches personal lives by fostering a deeper understanding of the world and contributing to a well-rounded and informed perspective.

Tips for Embracing Continuous Learning:

• Set Learning Goals: Define specific learning goals, both short-term and long-term. This provides a sense of direction and purpose to your learning journey.

• Diversify Learning Sources: Explore a variety of learning sources, including books, online courses, workshops, webinars, podcasts, and mentorship. Diversifying your sources ensures a well-rounded education.

• Stay Inquisitive: Cultivate a curious mindset. Ask questions, seek answers, and remain open to exploring topics beyond your immediate field of expertise.

• Allocate Time for Learning: Dedicate regular time to learning activities. This could be a few hours per week for reading, taking courses, or engaging in hands-on learning experiences.

• Leverage Technology: Take advantage of online platforms, e-learning courses, and educational apps that provide convenient and accessible learning opportunities.

• Join Professional Networks: Participate in professional networks, forums, and communities where you can exchange ideas, learn from others, and stay updated on industry trends.

• Seek Feedback: Request feedback on your learning progress. Constructive feedback can provide valuable insights and guide your future learning endeavors.

• Document Your Learning: Keep a learning journal or portfolio to document your achievements, insights, and the skills you've acquired. This serves as a tangible record of your continuous learning journey.

• Embrace Failure as a Learning Opportunity: View setbacks and challenges as opportunities for learning and growth. Analyze what went wrong, adjust your approach, and apply the lessons learned.

• Attend Conferences and Workshops: Participate in conferences, workshops, and seminars related to your field or areas of interest. These events offer networking opportunities and exposure to the latest developments.

• Engage in Hands-On Projects: Apply your learning by working on practical projects. Hands-on experience reinforces theoretical knowledge and enhances your skills.

• Stay Current with Industry Trends: Stay informed about industry trends, emerging technologies, and relevant news. This knowledge helps you remain competitive in your field.

• Share Knowledge: Teach others what you've learned. Whether through mentoring, writing, or presenting, sharing your knowledge reinforces your understanding and contributes to the learning community.

• Celebrate Milestones: Celebrate your learning milestones, no matter how small. Recognizing your achievements motivates you to continue your learning journey.

Continuous learning is a powerful tool for personal and professional development. By adopting a mindset of lifelong learning and actively seeking opportunities to expand your knowledge and skills, you can stay adaptable, resilient, and ready to face the challenges and opportunities that come your way.

CHAPTER THREE

COGNITIVE ACTIVITIES

Cognitive activities are exercises and tasks that stimulate mental processes, enhance brain function, and promote overall cognitive health. Engaging in these activities can improve memory, attention, problem-solving skills, and cognitive abilities. Here are various cognitive activities that you can incorporate into your routine:

1. Puzzles and Games:

• Crossword Puzzles: Stimulate language and vocabulary skills.

• Sudoku: Enhance logical and numerical reasoning.

• Chess or Checkers: Boost strategic thinking and planning.

2. Memory Exercises:

• Memory Games: Play games that challenge memory recall, such as matching games or concentration.

• Flashcards: Create flashcards for learning new information or reinforcing existing knowledge.

3. Learning a New Skill:

• Language Learning: Mastering a new language enhances cognitive abilities.

• Musical Instrument: Learning to play an instrument engages various cognitive functions.

4. Reading and Writing:

• Reading Books: Explore a variety of genres to stimulate imagination and comprehension.

• Journaling: Expressing thoughts through writing helps with cognitive organization.

5. Brain-Training Apps:

• Lumosity, Elevate, or Peak: These apps offer a variety of cognitive exercises targeting memory, attention, and problem-solving.

6. Critical Thinking Exercises:

• Logic Puzzles: Challenge yourself with puzzles that require deductive reasoning.

• Debates or Discussions: Engage in conversations that require critical thinking and analysis.

7. Art and Creativity:

• Drawing or Painting: Enhance visual-spatial skills and creativity.

• Crafting: Activities like knitting or origami improve focus and coordination.

8. Mindfulness and Meditation:

• Mindfulness Practices: Techniques such as meditation and deep breathing contribute to overall cognitive well-being.

9. Online Courses:

• Platforms like Coursera or Khan Academy: Enroll in courses covering a wide range of topics for continuous learning.

10. Social Engagement:

• Socializing: Regular interactions with others support cognitive health.

• Join Clubs or Groups: Participate in groups related to your interests.

11. Strategy Games:

• Board Games: Games like Risk, Settlers of Catan, or Stratego promote strategic thinking.

• Online Strategy Games: Explore digital games that challenge problem-solving skills.

12. Math Challenges:

• Math Puzzles: Solve mathematical puzzles and challenges.

• Budgeting: Engage in financial planning and budgeting exercises.

13. Memory Techniques:

• Mnemonics: Use mnemonic devices to remember information more effectively.

• Chunking: Break down large amounts of information into smaller chunks for easier recall.

14. Physical Exercise:

• Aerobic Exercise: Regular physical activity has been linked to improved cognitive function.

• Yoga: Combines physical activity with mindfulness, benefiting both body and mind.

15. Cooking and Recipes:

• Following Recipes: Enhance sequential memory and attention to detail.

• Experimenting with Ingredients: Stimulate creativity and problem-solving.

16. Memory Strategies:

• Visualization: Create mental images to aid memory recall.

• Association: Connect new information with familiar concepts.

17. Educational Podcasts:

• Listen to Podcasts: Explore podcasts on a variety of educational topics to expand your knowledge.

18. Trivia and Quizzes:

• Trivia Nights: Participate in trivia games or quizzes that cover a range of subjects.

19. Travel and Exploration:

• Learning about Different Cultures: Expand your cultural knowledge through books, documentaries, or travel.

20. Problem-Solving Activities:

• Escape Room Games: Engage in activities that require teamwork and problem-solving.

• Riddles and Brainteasers: Challenge your brain with puzzles that require creative thinking.

Incorporating a variety of cognitive activities into your routine can provide holistic stimulation for your brain. Remember to choose activities that align with your interests and preferences to make the learning process enjoyable and sustainable.

Engaging in hobbies and creative pursuits is not only enjoyable but also essential for overall well-being. Hobbies provide a way to relax, unwind, and express oneself creatively. They contribute to mental health, help manage stress, and offer a sense of accomplishment. Here are various hobbies and creative pursuits that you can explore:

1. Artistic Hobbies:

• Drawing and Sketching: Express your creativity through visual art.

• Painting: Explore different painting mediums, such as watercolors, acrylics, or oils.

• Photography: Capture moments and scenes that inspire you.

2. Crafting:

• Knitting or Crocheting: Create handmade items like scarves, blankets, or clothing.

• Origami: Master the art of paper folding.

• DIY Projects: Engage in do-it-yourself projects, from home decor to handmade gifts.

3. Writing:

• Journaling: Express your thoughts, feelings, and experiences.

• Creative Writing: Explore short stories, poetry, or novel writing.

• Blogging: Share your interests or expertise through online platforms.

4. Music:

• Playing an Instrument: Learn to play a musical instrument, whether it's the guitar, piano, or any other.

• Singing: Join a choir or simply sing for enjoyment.

5. Cooking and Baking:

• Experimenting with Recipes: Try new cuisines or create your own recipes.

• Cake Decorating: Learn the art of decorating cakes and pastries.

6. Gardening:

• Planting and Tending to a Garden: Grow flowers, herbs, or vegetables.

• Indoor Plants: Care for indoor plants and create a green space at home.

7. Outdoor Activities:

• Hiking: Explore nature trails and enjoy the outdoors.

• Cycling: Take up cycling for both exercise and leisure.

• Bird Watching: Observe and identify different bird species.

8. Reading:

• Book Club Participation: Join a book club to discuss literature with others.

• Genre Exploration: Explore different genres to expand your reading interests.

9. Fitness and Wellness:

• Yoga or Pilates: Improve flexibility and mindfulness.

• Dance: Take dance classes or dance at home for fitness and fun.

• Martial Arts: Learn self-defense and discipline through martial arts.

10. Board Games and Puzzles:

• Board Game Nights: Play board games with friends or family.

• Jigsaw Puzzles: Engage in the challenge of completing puzzles.

11. Travel and Exploration:

• Travel Photography: Combine travel with photography to document your adventures.

• Collecting Souvenirs: Collect souvenirs from different places you visit.

12. Astronomy:

• Stargazing: Learn about constellations and explore the night sky.

• Telescope Observation: Invest in a telescope for a closer look at celestial bodies.

13. Model Building:

• Model Cars, Planes, or Ships: Assemble and paint model kits.

• LEGO Building: Create intricate structures and designs with LEGO sets.

14. Learning a New Language:

• Language Apps: Use language-learning apps to acquire a new language.

• Language Classes: Enroll in formal language classes for in-depth learning.

15. Collecting:

• Stamp Collecting: Explore the world of philately.

• Coin Collecting: Collect coins from different regions or historical periods.

16. Mindfulness and Meditation:

• Mindfulness Practices: Engage in mindfulness meditation or relaxation techniques.

• Breathing Exercises: Incorporate deep breathing exercises for relaxation.

17. Film and Cinema:

• Film Critique: Watch and analyze films, exploring different genres and directors.

• Filmmaking: Try your hand at making short films or videos.

18. Home Improvement:

• DIY Home Projects: Renovate or redecorate areas of your home.

• Furniture Restoration: Restore or repurpose old furniture.

19. Historical Exploration:

• Genealogy Research: Explore your family history and create a family tree.

- Visit Historical Sites: Learn about history by visiting museums and historical landmarks.

20. Virtual Reality (VR) Gaming:

- VR Experiences: Explore virtual reality for gaming and interactive experiences.

Choosing a hobby or creative pursuit that aligns with your interests and passions can provide a sense of fulfillment and joy. Remember that the goal is to enjoy the process, express yourself, and create a balance that enhances your overall well-being.

IMPORTANCE OF SOCIALIZING

Socializing, or engaging in social activities and interactions with others, holds significant importance for mental, emotional, and even physical well-being. Human beings are inherently social creatures, and our relationships and connections with others play a crucial role in shaping our overall quality of life. Here are several key reasons highlighting the importance of socializing:

1. Mental and Emotional Health:

• Reduced Stress: Socializing provides an opportunity to share experiences, express emotions, and receive emotional support, which can help alleviate stress.

• Enhanced Mood: Positive social interactions release hormones like oxytocin and serotonin, contributing to improved mood and a sense of well-being.

• Prevention of Mental Health Issues: Regular social engagement is associated with a lower risk of mental health issues such as depression and anxiety.

2. Cognitive Benefits:

• Stimulated Brain Function: Socializing stimulates the brain, challenging cognitive functions and contributing to mental agility.

• Intellectual Stimulation: Engaging in conversations, debates, or discussions exposes individuals to diverse perspectives, fostering intellectual growth.

3. Sense of Belonging:

• Community and Connection: Socializing helps individuals feel a sense of belonging to a community, family, or social group.

• Reduced Isolation: Regular social interactions reduce feelings of loneliness and isolation, which can have negative effects on mental health.

4. Emotional Support:

• Friendship and Companionship: Socializing allows for the development of friendships and meaningful relationships that offer emotional support during both good and challenging times.

• Validation and Understanding: Sharing experiences with others provides validation and understanding, reducing feelings of isolation.

5. Improved Communication Skills:

• Enhanced Verbal and Non-Verbal Communication: Regular socializing hones communication skills, both in expressing oneself and understanding others.

• Conflict Resolution: Social interactions provide opportunities to practice conflict resolution and negotiation skills.

6. Physical Health Benefits:

• Stress Reduction: Socializing contributes to lower stress levels, which, in turn, positively impacts physical health.

• Increased Immune Function: Positive social connections have been linked to improved immune system function.

• Longevity: Strong social ties are associated with increased life expectancy.

7. Networking and Professional Growth:

• Career Opportunities: Socializing in professional settings facilitates networking, which can lead to career opportunities, collaborations, and professional growth.

• Team Building: Social interactions within the workplace contribute to effective team building and collaboration.

8. Skill Development:

• Interpersonal Skills: Socializing helps develop interpersonal skills, including empathy, active listening, and conflict resolution.

• Adaptability: Interacting with diverse groups of people enhances adaptability and the ability to navigate different social situations.

9. Quality of Life:

• Enjoyment and Fulfillment: Socializing adds joy and fulfillment to life, creating memorable experiences and positive memories.

• Shared Activities: Engaging in social activities allows individuals to share hobbies, interests, and experiences with others.

10. Support Systems in Times of Need:

• Crisis Support: Social connections provide a support system during challenging times, offering practical help and emotional assistance.

• Coping Mechanism: Socializing can be a healthy coping mechanism, aiding in resilience and recovery during difficult periods.

11. Learning and Growth:

• Exposure to Different Perspectives: Socializing exposes individuals to diverse viewpoints and cultures, contributing to personal growth and a broader understanding of the world.

• Continuous Learning: Engaging in conversations with others allows for the exchange of ideas and knowledge.

12. Happiness and Well-Being:

• Positive Relationships: Strong social connections contribute significantly to overall happiness and life satisfaction.

• Shared Joy: Celebrating successes and joys with others amplifies the positive experiences in life.

In summary, socializing is a fundamental aspect of human life that contributes to mental, emotional, and physical well-being. Whether through family, friends, colleagues, or community involvement, fostering positive social connections is an investment in one's health, happiness, and overall quality of life.

BUILDING AND MAINTAINING RELATIONSHIPS

Building and maintaining healthy relationships is essential for overall well-being and fulfillment. Strong connections with family, friends, colleagues, and romantic partners contribute significantly to emotional and mental health. Here are key principles and tips for building and maintaining positive relationships:

Building Relationships:

Open Communication:

• Active Listening: Practice active listening to understand others' perspectives and feelings.

• Express Yourself Clearly: Communicate openly and honestly, expressing your thoughts and emotions clearly.

Mutual Respect:

• Value Differences: Respect and appreciate the unique qualities and differences in others.

• Boundaries: Establish and respect personal boundaries within the relationship.

Trust:

• Reliability: Be consistent and reliable, keeping promises and commitments.

• Transparency: Foster trust through openness and transparency in communication.

Quality Time:

• Invest Time: Prioritize spending quality time together to build shared experiences.

• Meaningful Activities: Engage in activities that both parties enjoy and find meaningful.

Support and Empathy:

• Empathize: Understand and empathize with others' feelings and experiences.

• Provide Support: Offer emotional support during both good and challenging times.

Shared Goals and Values:

• Discuss Goals: Align on shared goals and values to build a sense of purpose.

• Celebrate Achievements: Celebrate individual and shared accomplishments.

Positive Communication:

• Use Positive Language: Frame discussions in a positive manner, focusing on solutions rather than blame.

• Avoid Assumptions: Clarify information to prevent misunderstandings and assumptions.

Apologize and Forgive:

• Apologize Sincerely: Offer sincere apologies when needed, taking responsibility for mistakes.

• Forgive: Practice forgiveness to let go of resentment and move forward.

Maintaining Relationships:

Consistent Communication:

• Regular Check-Ins: Schedule regular check-ins to discuss the state of the relationship and address concerns.

• Express Appreciation: Regularly express gratitude and appreciation for each other.

Adaptability:

• Flexibility: Be adaptable to changes and challenges, adjusting expectations as needed.

• Continuous Growth: Embrace the idea that relationships require ongoing effort and growth.

Conflict Resolution:

• Healthy Conflict Resolution: Address conflicts with respect and a focus on finding solutions.

• Seek Common Ground: Identify areas of agreement and work towards compromise.

Independence and Space:

• Maintain Independence: Foster individual interests and pursuits outside the relationship.

• Respect Personal Space: Allow each other personal space and time for self-reflection.

Shared Responsibilities:

• Equitable Distribution: Share responsibilities and collaborate on tasks to create a sense of partnership.

• Open Communication about Roles: Discuss and openly communicate about expectations and roles within the relationship.

Cultivate Intimacy:

• Emotional Intimacy: Nurture emotional intimacy through open and vulnerable communication.

• Physical Intimacy: Maintain physical affection and closeness to strengthen the bond.

Celebrate Milestones:

• Anniversaries and Achievements: Acknowledge and celebrate relationship milestones and individual achievements.

• Create Rituals: Establish meaningful rituals and traditions to reinforce connection.

Regular Evaluation:

• Reflect and Evaluate: Periodically reflect on the state of the relationship and evaluate areas for improvement.

• Set Relationship Goals: Set realistic goals for the relationship and work towards them together.

Show Appreciation:

• Express Gratitude: Regularly express gratitude for the positive aspects of the relationship.

• Small Gestures: Show appreciation through small gestures and acts of kindness.

Quality Time:

• Prioritize Quality Time: Continue to prioritize spending quality time together, even amidst busy schedules.

• Adventures and Exploration: Engage in new activities and adventures to keep the relationship dynamic.

Weathering Challenges:

• Facing Challenges Together: Approach challenges as a team, supporting each other through difficult times.

• Seeking Help: If needed, be open to seeking professional help or counseling during challenging periods.

Building and maintaining healthy relationships is an ongoing process that requires effort, communication, and a commitment to mutual growth. By incorporating these principles into your interactions, you can create and sustain meaningful connections that contribute to a fulfilling and supportive life.

HEALTHY BOUNDARIES

Establishing and maintaining healthy boundaries is essential for cultivating positive relationships, maintaining well-being, and fostering personal growth. Healthy boundaries create a framework that defines acceptable behavior, protects individual autonomy, and promotes mutual respect. Here are key principles and tips for setting and maintaining healthy boundaries:

Understanding Healthy Boundaries:

Self-Awareness:

• Know Your Limits: Understand your emotional, physical, and mental limits.

• Identify Values: Clarify your values and what is important to you in relationships.

Clear Communication:

• Express Needs Clearly: Clearly communicate your needs, expectations, and limits.

• Use "I" Statements: Frame your boundaries using "I" statements to express your feelings and preferences without sounding accusatory.

Consistency:

• Be Consistent: Establish consistent boundaries and enforce them across different situations.

• Avoid Mixed Messages: Consistency helps avoid confusion and ensures others understand your expectations.

Respect for Others:

• Respect Others' Boundaries: Extend the same respect for others' boundaries that you expect for your own.

• Active Listening: Listen actively to understand and respect the boundaries communicated by others.

Tips for Setting Healthy Boundaries:

Know Your Limits:

• Recognize Warning Signs: Be aware of situations or behaviors that make you uncomfortable or trigger stress.

• Prioritize Self-Care: Prioritize self-care activities to maintain your physical and mental well-being.

Learn to Say No:

• Be Assertive: Practice assertiveness in saying no when necessary.

• Avoid Overcommitting: Resist the urge to overcommit by setting realistic expectations for your time and energy.

Identify Your Values:

• Clarify Core Values: Clearly understand your core values, guiding principles, and priorities.

• Align Boundaries with Values: Ensure that your boundaries align with your values and principles.

Communicate Clearly:

• Use Direct Communication: Clearly communicate your expectations, preferences, and limits directly.

• Avoid Ambiguity: Be specific about what is acceptable and what is not.

Understand Emotional Boundaries:

• Recognize Emotional Needs: Understand your emotional needs and communicate them to others.

• Establish Emotional Space: Set boundaries around emotional space and avoid excessive emotional dependency.

Be Flexible:

• Adapt to Situations: Recognize that boundaries may need to be adjusted based on different situations.

• Consider Others' Perspectives: Be open to understanding others' perspectives and finding common ground.

Seek Support:

• Consult Trusted Individuals: Seek advice from trusted friends, family, or mentors when navigating complex boundary issues.

• Therapeutic Support: Consider therapy or counseling for guidance in setting and maintaining healthy boundaries.

Maintaining Healthy Boundaries:

Consistent Enforcement:

• Enforce Boundaries Firmly: Reinforce your boundaries consistently, even when faced with resistance or pushback.

• Avoid Guilt: Resist feelings of guilt when enforcing boundaries that prioritize your well-being.

Monitor Relationships:

• Assess Relationships Periodically: Regularly evaluate the health of your relationships and whether boundaries are being respected.

• Address Violations Promptly: Address boundary violations promptly to prevent patterns of disrespect.

Self-Reflection:

• Regular Self-Reflection: Periodically reflect on your own boundaries and assess whether they align with your evolving needs.

• Learn from Experiences: Learn from experiences, especially situations where boundaries were tested or violated.

Empower Others:

• Encourage Others' Boundaries: Encourage and respect the boundaries of others in your relationships.

• Create Empowering Environments: Foster environments where everyone feels empowered to express their needs.

Seek Feedback:

• Request Feedback: Seek feedback from trusted individuals on your ability to maintain healthy boundaries.

• Open Communication: Encourage open communication about boundaries in your relationships.

Adapt to Changes:

• Adapt to Life Changes: Be flexible and willing to adjust your boundaries as life circumstances and relationships evolve.

• Communication in Changes: Communicate changes in your boundaries clearly to those affected.

Remember that setting and maintaining healthy boundaries is an ongoing process that requires self-awareness, assertiveness, and effective communication. Prioritizing your well-being while respecting the needs of others contributes to the creation of balanced and positive relationships.

CHAPTER FOUR

IMPORTANCE OF REGULAR CHECK-UPS AND SCREENINGS

Regular check-ups and screenings are crucial components of preventive healthcare that play a significant role in maintaining overall well-being and detecting potential health issues early on. Here are several reasons highlighting the importance of regular check-ups and screenings:

1. Early Detection of Health Issues:

• Cancer Screening: Regular screenings, such as mammograms, Pap smears, and colonoscopies, can detect cancer at early, more treatable stages.

• Blood Pressure Checks: Monitoring blood pressure helps identify hypertension early, reducing the risk of heart disease and stroke.

• Blood Tests: Routine blood tests can detect conditions like diabetes, high cholesterol, and anemia before symptoms manifest.

2. Prevention and Risk Reduction:

• Vaccinations: Routine vaccinations protect against preventable diseases and contribute to public health by reducing the spread of infectious agents.

• Behavioral Counseling: Regular check-ups provide opportunities for healthcare professionals to offer advice on lifestyle changes, diet, exercise, and smoking cessation to prevent health problems.

3. Management of Chronic Conditions:

• Monitoring Chronic Diseases: For individuals with chronic conditions like diabetes or hypertension, regular check-ups help monitor disease progression and adjust treatment plans as needed.

• Medication Management: Healthcare providers can assess medication effectiveness, address side effects, and make adjustments during check-ups.

4. Health Education and Promotion:

• Wellness Counseling: Healthcare professionals provide guidance on healthy living, stress management, and preventive measures during check-ups.

• Risk Assessment: Individuals receive personalized risk assessments, helping them understand potential health risks and take proactive steps to mitigate them.

5. Mental Health Screening:

• Mental Health Assessment: Regular check-ups include discussions about mental health, allowing for the identification of mental health concerns and the provision of appropriate support.

• Access to Resources: Check-ups provide an opportunity for individuals to access mental health resources, counseling, or therapy.

6. Monitoring Growth and Development:

• Pediatric Check-ups: Regular pediatric check-ups monitor children's growth, development, and milestones, allowing for early intervention if developmental issues arise.

• Adolescent Health: Check-ups for adolescents address specific health concerns related to puberty, mental health, and lifestyle choices.

7. Establishing Baseline Health Data:

• Health Records: Regular check-ups contribute to maintaining comprehensive health records, allowing healthcare providers to establish baseline data for each individual.

• Tracking Changes Over Time: Baseline data facilitates the tracking of changes in health status over time, aiding in the early identification of abnormalities.

8. Long-Term Health Maintenance:

• Aging Population: Regular check-ups become increasingly important as individuals age, assisting in the detection and management of age-related conditions.

• Preventive Care for Older Adults: Health screenings for conditions like osteoporosis, vision problems, and cognitive decline become more critical for older adults.

9. Patient-Provider Relationship:

• Trust and Communication: Regular check-ups foster trust and open communication between patients and healthcare providers.

• Patient Engagement: Patients who engage in regular check-ups are more likely to actively participate in their healthcare decisions and follow preventive recommendations.

10. Cost-Effective Healthcare:

• Preventive vs. Reactive Care: Preventive care is often more cost-effective than reactive care, as early detection and intervention can reduce the financial burden of treating advanced illnesses.

• Avoiding Emergency Care: Regular check-ups can help identify and address health issues before they escalate to the point of requiring emergency care.

11. Compliance with Guidelines:

• Adherence to Screening Guidelines: Regular check-ups ensure adherence to established screening guidelines, which are based on age, gender, family history, and risk factors.

• Customized Preventive Care: Healthcare providers can tailor preventive care recommendations based on individual needs and risk factors.

12. Public Health Impact:

• Disease Surveillance: Regular check-ups contribute to disease surveillance and monitoring, providing valuable data for public health initiatives and research.

• Population Health Management: Identifying and addressing health issues at the population level helps manage and improve overall community health.

In summary, regular check-ups and screenings are proactive measures that contribute to preventive healthcare, early detection of health issues, and the promotion of overall well-being. By investing in routine healthcare visits, individuals can actively manage their health, reduce the risk of serious conditions, and enhance their quality of life.

VACCINATIONS AND IMMUNIZATIONS

Vaccinations and immunizations are essential components of preventive healthcare that help protect individuals and communities from a range of infectious diseases. Here are key points outlining the importance and benefits of vaccinations:

1. Prevention of Serious Illnesses:

• Disease Prevention: Vaccinations are designed to prevent the onset of serious and potentially life-threatening diseases caused by viruses and bacteria.

• Eradication of Diseases: Successful vaccination programs have led to the eradication or significant reduction of certain diseases, such as smallpox.

2. Herd Immunity:

• Community Protection: Vaccinations contribute to herd immunity, where a sufficient percentage of the population is immune to a disease, reducing its spread and protecting those who cannot be vaccinated.

• Protecting Vulnerable Populations: Herd immunity is particularly important for protecting individuals with weakened immune systems, infants, and the elderly who may be more susceptible to severe complications.

3. Effective Public Health Strategy:

• Disease Control: Vaccination is a highly effective public health strategy for controlling and preventing the spread of infectious diseases.

• Reduction of Outbreaks: Vaccination programs help prevent outbreaks and minimize the impact of diseases on communities.

4. Safe and Well-Regulated:

• Stringent Testing: Vaccines undergo rigorous testing and monitoring for safety and efficacy before being approved for use.

• Continuous Monitoring: Post-marketing surveillance ensures ongoing monitoring of vaccine safety, allowing for prompt response to any potential concerns.

5. Cost-Effective Health Intervention:

• Prevention of Healthcare Costs: Vaccination is a cost-effective way to prevent illnesses and reduce the economic burden associated with treating infectious diseases.

• Avoidance of Complications: Vaccines help prevent complications that may require extensive medical treatment and hospitalization.

6. Protection Across the Lifespan:

• Childhood Vaccines: Immunizations in childhood protect against diseases like measles, mumps, rubella, polio, and pertussis.

• Adult Vaccines: Vaccination remains important throughout adulthood to protect against diseases such as influenza, pneumonia, and shingles.

7. Global Health Impact:

• Global Disease Control: Vaccination programs contribute to global efforts in controlling and eliminating infectious diseases worldwide.

• Global Collaboration: International vaccination initiatives promote collaboration and support for countries with limited healthcare resources.

8. Reduced Antibiotic Resistance:

• Prevention of Bacterial Infections: Vaccines can prevent bacterial infections, reducing the need for antibiotics and helping to combat antibiotic resistance.

• Avoidance of Secondary Infections: By preventing primary infections, vaccines indirectly contribute to the reduction of secondary bacterial infections.

9. Improved Quality of Life:

• Prevention of Disability: Vaccinations prevent illnesses that may lead to long-term disabilities or chronic health conditions.

• Enhanced Well-Being: Immunization contributes to an improved quality of life by reducing the burden of preventable diseases.

10. Responsiveness to Emerging Threats:

• Rapid Development: Advances in vaccine technology allow for the rapid development of vaccines in response to emerging infectious threats, such as new strains of influenza or novel viruses.

• Pandemic Preparedness: Vaccination plays a crucial role in preparedness for potential pandemics, providing a proactive approach to mitigating the impact of emerging infectious diseases.

11. Individual and Collective Responsibility:

• Protecting Self and Others: Vaccination is an individual responsibility to protect oneself and contribute to the collective effort in safeguarding public health.

• Ethical Considerations: Vaccination reflects a commitment to the well-being of both oneself and the broader community.

12. Public Confidence in Healthcare:

• Trust in Medical Advances: Successful vaccination programs contribute to public trust in medical science and advancements in healthcare.

• Community Confidence: High vaccination rates foster community confidence in the effectiveness of preventive measures against infectious diseases.

In conclusion, vaccinations and immunizations are vital tools in preventing the spread of infectious diseases, protecting individuals and communities, and promoting global health. By actively participating in vaccination programs, individuals contribute to the well-being of both themselves and the broader

Health monitoring and self-exams are proactive approaches to maintaining one's well-being by regularly assessing various aspects of health and detecting potential issues early. These practices empower individuals to take an active role in their health management. Here are key components and benefits of health monitoring and self-exams:

1. Regular Health Check-ups:

• Scheduled Check-ups: Periodic visits to healthcare professionals for routine check-ups enable the monitoring of overall health.

• Early Detection: Regular check-ups can help detect health issues at an early stage when they are often more treatable.

2. Self-Exams for Early Detection:

• Breast Self-Exam: Regular breast self-exams can help identify changes or abnormalities that may require further evaluation.

• Testicular Self-Exam: Men can perform testicular self-exams to detect abnormalities that may indicate potential issues.

3. Monitoring Vital Signs:

• Blood Pressure Monitoring: Regular monitoring of blood pressure helps identify hypertension and reduces the risk of cardiovascular diseases.

• Heart Rate and Pulse Monitoring: Tracking heart rate and pulse can provide insights into cardiovascular health.

4. Blood Glucose Monitoring:

• Diabetes Management: Individuals with diabetes can monitor blood glucose levels regularly to manage their condition effectively.

• Preventive Measures: Monitoring blood glucose levels may help prevent complications associated with diabetes.

5. Body Weight and Composition:

• Regular Weighing: Tracking body weight can help manage weight-related issues and promote a healthy lifestyle.

• Body Composition Measurements: Assessing body fat percentage and muscle mass provides a more comprehensive understanding of overall health.

6. Skin Checks:

• Skin Self-Exams: Regular skin checks help identify changes in moles or skin conditions that may require attention.

• Sun Protection: Monitoring the skin for changes helps prevent skin cancers and other sun-related issues.

7. Dental Health Monitoring:

• Regular Dental Check-ups: Routine dental exams are essential for maintaining oral health and preventing dental issues.

• Oral Hygiene Practices: Daily monitoring of oral hygiene, including brushing and flossing, contributes to overall dental well-being.

8. Eye Health Checks:

• Regular Eye Exams: Routine eye exams can detect vision problems, eye diseases, and other issues affecting eye health.

• Screen Time Management: Monitoring screen time and taking breaks can reduce eye strain and promote eye health.

9. Mental Health Self-Assessment:

• Self-Reflection: Regular self-reflection helps assess mental well-being and identify signs of stress, anxiety, or depression.

• Seeking Support: Recognizing changes in mental health early allows for timely intervention and seeking support when needed.

10. Bone Health Monitoring:

• Bone Density Scans: In certain populations, monitoring bone density through scans can help prevent osteoporosis and fractures.

• Calcium and Vitamin D Intake: Maintaining adequate calcium and vitamin D intake supports bone health.

11. Gastrointestinal Health Monitoring:

• Dietary Habits: Monitoring dietary habits aids in digestive health and may prevent issues like indigestion and constipation.

• Colon Cancer Screening: Regular screenings, such as colonoscopies, contribute to the early detection of colorectal cancer.

12. Reproductive Health Checks:

• Menstrual Cycle Monitoring: Regular tracking of menstrual cycles helps women understand their reproductive health.

• Sexual Health Exams: Routine screenings for sexually transmitted infections contribute to reproductive health.

13. Immunization Status:

• Vaccination Record: Keeping track of vaccination records ensures that individuals stay up-to-date on immunizations.

• Preventive Health Measures: Immunizations play a crucial role in preventing certain infectious diseases.

14. Health Monitoring Apps:

• Fitness Trackers: Wearable devices and apps can monitor physical activity, sleep patterns, and overall fitness.

• Health Apps: Apps that track nutrition, medication adherence, and mental well-being provide valuable insights.

15. Regular Exercise Routine:

• Physical Activity Monitoring: Regular exercise contributes to overall health, promoting cardiovascular fitness, strength, and flexibility.

• Preventive Benefits: Physical activity is associated with a reduced risk of various chronic diseases.

16. Financial Health Assessment:

• Financial Check-up: Monitoring financial health helps reduce stress and promotes overall well-being.

• Budgeting: Regularly assessing financial habits and creating budgets contribute to financial stability.

17. Sleep Hygiene Practices:

• Sleep Patterns Observation: Monitoring sleep patterns and quality helps identify potential sleep disorders.

• Sleep Hygiene: Practicing good sleep hygiene contributes to better overall health and well-being.

18. Allergies and Sensitivities:

• Food Diary: Keeping a food diary helps identify and manage food allergies or sensitivities.

• Environmental Triggers: Identifying and avoiding environmental triggers contributes to allergy management.

19. Posture and Ergonomics:

• Posture Assessment: Monitoring and maintaining good posture contribute to musculoskeletal health.

• Ergonomic Practices: Ensuring ergonomic workspaces reduces the risk of musculoskeletal issues.

20. Hydration Status:

• Fluid Intake Monitoring: Staying adequately hydrated supports overall health and helps prevent dehydration-related issues.

• Urine Color Observation: Monitoring urine color is an easy way to assess hydration levels.

Benefits of Health Monitoring and Self-Exams:

• Early Intervention: Early detection of health issues allows for timely intervention and treatment.

• Empowerment: Individuals are empowered to actively participate in their health management.

• Preventive Focus: Monitoring supports a preventive approach to health, reducing the risk of complications.

• Improved Quality of Life: Proactive health monitoring contributes to an improved quality of life and overall well-being.

Incorporating health monitoring and self-exams into one's routine contributes to a holistic and proactive approach to well-being, fostering a sense of empowerment and allowing for early detection and intervention when needed.

Avoidance of harmful substances is a critical aspect of maintaining good health and well-being. Harmful substances can have adverse effects on various aspects of health, including physical, mental, and social well-being. Here are key reasons and strategies for avoiding harmful substances:

1. Tobacco and Smoking:

• Health Risks: Smoking is a major cause of preventable diseases, including lung cancer, heart disease, and respiratory issues.

• Strategies: Avoid tobacco products, seek smoking cessation programs, and create smoke-free environments.

2. Excessive Alcohol Consumption:

• Liver Damage: Heavy alcohol consumption can lead to liver cirrhosis and other organ damage.

• Strategies: Limit alcohol intake, know personal limits, and seek help if struggling with alcohol dependence.

3. Illicit Drugs:

• Addiction and Health Risks: Illicit drugs can lead to addiction, mental health issues, and severe physical harm.

• Strategies: Avoid recreational drug use, seek support for addiction, and engage in drug education programs.

4. Prescription Drug Abuse:

• Dependency and Health Risks: Misuse of prescription drugs can lead to dependency and various health risks.

• Strategies: Use prescription medications as prescribed, communicate openly with healthcare providers, and properly dispose of unused medications.

5. Unhealthy Diet:

• Nutritional Deficiencies: Consuming excessive processed foods, sugary drinks, and unhealthy fats can lead to nutritional deficiencies and obesity.

• Strategies: Adopt a balanced and nutritious diet, limit processed foods, and stay hydrated.

6. Lack of Physical Activity:

• Chronic Diseases: Sedentary lifestyles contribute to the development of chronic diseases and overall poor health.

• Strategies: Incorporate regular physical activity into daily routines, such as walking, jogging, or engaging in sports.

7. Environmental Toxins:

• Respiratory and Health Issues: Exposure to environmental pollutants, chemicals, and toxins can lead to respiratory problems and other health issues.

• Strategies: Minimize exposure to environmental toxins, use eco-friendly products, and support environmental conservation efforts.

8. Poor Sleep Habits:

• Sleep Disorders: Inadequate sleep or poor sleep quality can contribute to various health problems, including impaired cognitive function.

• Strategies: Prioritize good sleep hygiene, establish consistent sleep patterns, and create a comfortable sleep environment.

9. Excessive Screen Time:

• Eye Strain and Sleep Disruption: Excessive screen time can lead to eye strain, disrupted sleep patterns, and sedentary behavior.

• Strategies: Implement screen time limits, take breaks, and practice the 20-20-20 rule for eye health.

10. Stress and Burnout:

• Mental Health Impact: Chronic stress and burnout can have profound effects on mental health and overall well-being.

• Strategies: Practice stress management techniques, prioritize self-care, and seek support when needed.

11. Unsafe Sexual Practices:

• Sexually Transmitted Infections (STIs): Engaging in unsafe sexual practices can lead to the transmission of STIs.

• Strategies: Use protection, practice safe sex, and communicate openly with sexual partners.

12. Inadequate Hydration:

• Dehydration: Insufficient water intake can lead to dehydration, impacting physical and cognitive functions.

• Strategies: Drink an adequate amount of water daily, especially in hot or humid conditions.

13. Sun Exposure Without Protection:

• Skin Damage: Prolonged sun exposure without protection can lead to skin damage, including sunburn and an increased risk of skin cancer.

• Strategies: Use sunscreen, wear protective clothing, and avoid excessive sun exposure, especially during peak hours.

14. Inadequate Dental Hygiene:

• Oral Health Issues: Poor dental hygiene can lead to issues such as cavities, gum disease, and bad breath.

• Strategies: Brush and floss regularly, attend dental check-ups, and maintain good oral hygiene practices.

15. Exposure to Secondhand Smoke:

• Respiratory Issues: Inhaling secondhand smoke can lead to respiratory issues and increase the risk of certain health conditions.

• Strategies: Avoid exposure to secondhand smoke, especially in enclosed spaces.

16. Lack of Mental Health Support:

• Psychological Strain: Ignoring mental health needs and lacking a support system can lead to emotional strain.

• Strategies: Seek professional help when needed, maintain strong social connections, and prioritize mental well-being.

17. Lack of Safety Measures:

• Accidents and Injuries: Ignoring safety measures can lead to accidents and injuries.

• Strategies: Follow safety guidelines, use protective gear, and practice caution in various environments.

18. Overconsumption of Sugar:

• Metabolic Issues: Excessive sugar intake is linked to obesity, type 2 diabetes, and other metabolic issues.

• Strategies: Limit added sugar intake, read food labels, and choose natural sweeteners in moderation.

19. Overreliance on Technology:

• Social Isolation and Mental Health: Overreliance on technology can contribute to social isolation and impact mental health.

• Strategies: Balance technology use with face-to-face interactions, set boundaries, and engage in offline activities.

20. Lack of Vaccination:

• Vaccine-Preventable Diseases: Avoiding vaccinations can lead to the spread of preventable infectious diseases.

• Strategies: Stay up-to-date on recommended vaccinations and participate in public health vaccination programs.

In summary, avoiding harmful substances and adopting healthy lifestyle practices contribute significantly to overall well-being. It requires conscious efforts, informed choices, and a commitment to prioritizing health at various levels — physical, mental, and environmental. By avoiding harmful substances and embracing health-promoting behaviors, individuals can enhance their quality of life and reduce the risk of various health issues.

REGULAR HEALTH ASSESSMENTS AND GOAL SETTING

Regular health assessments and goal setting are integral components of proactive healthcare, enabling individuals to monitor their well-being, identify potential risk factors, and establish targeted objectives for improvement. Here's a breakdown of the importance, key elements, and benefits of regular health assessments and goal setting:

Importance of Regular Health Assessments:

Early Detection of Health Issues:

- Regular assessments facilitate the early detection of health issues, allowing for prompt intervention and treatment.

• Screenings and tests can identify risk factors for conditions like cardiovascular diseases, diabetes, and certain cancers.

Baseline Health Information:

• Establishing baseline health data through assessments provides a reference point for tracking changes over time.

• Comprehensive health information assists healthcare professionals in personalized care planning.

Preventive Healthcare:

• Health assessments focus on preventive measures, empowering individuals to adopt healthy lifestyles and behaviors.

• Vaccinations, screenings, and lifestyle counseling contribute to disease prevention.

Holistic Well-Being:

• Assessments consider various aspects of health, including physical, mental, and social well-being.

• Holistic evaluations address both immediate health concerns and potential long-term risks.

Physical Health Assessment:

• Measurements such as blood pressure, cholesterol levels, and body mass index (BMI) provide insights into cardiovascular health.

• Regular check-ups with healthcare providers assess overall physical well-being.

Mental Health Assessment:

• Screenings for mental health conditions, stress levels, and mood disorders are crucial for overall well-being.

• Open communication with healthcare professionals about mental health concerns is essential.

Lifestyle and Behavioral Assessments:

• Evaluating lifestyle factors, including diet, exercise, sleep, and substance use, helps identify areas for improvement.

• Behavioral assessments address habits that impact health, such as smoking, alcohol consumption, and physical activity.

Screenings and Tests:

• Routine screenings for conditions such as cancer, diabetes, and sexually transmitted infections (STIs) are essential.

• Age-appropriate tests, like mammograms and colonoscopies, contribute to early detection and prevention.

Vaccination Review:

• Ensuring up-to-date vaccinations protects against preventable infectious diseases.

• Regular reviews with healthcare providers help determine needed vaccinations based on age and risk factors.

Importance of Goal Setting:

Individualized Health Improvement:

• Goal setting allows individuals to tailor health improvement strategies to their unique needs and preferences.

• Personalized goals enhance motivation and engagement in the health improvement process.

Measurable Progress:

• Establishing measurable goals provides a clear framework for tracking progress.

• Achieving small milestones encourages ongoing commitment to health improvement.

Behavioral Change:

• Goals facilitate behavioral change by breaking down larger objectives into manageable, actionable steps.

• Specific and realistic goals are more likely to lead to sustainable lifestyle changes.

Preventive Health Maintenance:

• Goal setting supports ongoing preventive health efforts, ensuring individuals consistently prioritize well-being.

• Regularly reviewing and updating goals promotes continuous health improvement.

Elements of Effective Goal Setting:

Specific and Measurable Objectives:

• Goals should be specific, measurable, achievable, relevant, and time-bound (SMART).

• Clearly defined objectives provide a roadmap for health improvement.

Realistic and Attainable Targets:

• Setting realistic goals increases the likelihood of success and prevents discouragement.

• Small, achievable targets contribute to sustained motivation.

Incorporation of Healthy Habits:

• Goals should focus on adopting and maintaining healthy habits, such as regular exercise, balanced nutrition, and adequate sleep.

• Addressing specific lifestyle changes contributes to overall health improvement.

Regular Monitoring and Adjustments:

• Regularly monitor progress toward goals and be willing to adjust them based on changing circumstances or health status.

• Continuous assessment ensures goals remain relevant and achievable.

Support Systems and Accountability:

• Engage support systems, including healthcare professionals, family, and friends.

• Accountability mechanisms, such as tracking progress or sharing goals, enhance commitment.

Benefits of Regular Health Assessments and Goal Setting:

Proactive Health Management:

• Regular assessments empower individuals to take a proactive approach to their health.

• Identifying potential health risks early allows for timely interventions and preventive measures.

Enhanced Motivation:

• Goal setting enhances motivation by providing a clear vision of health improvement.

• Celebrating achievements, even small ones, boosts morale and encourages sustained efforts.

Long-Term Well-Being:

• Consistent health assessments and goal setting contribute to long-term well-being.

• Establishing healthy habits and maintaining preventive measures enhance overall health outcomes.

Informed Decision-Making:

• Regular assessments provide individuals with the information needed to make informed decisions about their health.

• Informed choices contribute to a proactive and engaged approach to healthcare.

Reduced Healthcare Costs:

• Early detection and prevention through regular assessments can lead to reduced healthcare costs.

• Proactively addressing health concerns may mitigate the need for more extensive and costly interventions.

In conclusion, regular health assessments and goal setting are integral components of a comprehensive and proactive healthcare strategy. By actively participating in assessments, setting realistic goals, and making informed decisions, individuals can optimize their well-being and work toward achieving and maintaining a healthier lifestyle.

CHAPTER FIVE

HOW TO CARRY OUT SUN SAFETY

Practicing sun safety is crucial for protecting your skin from harmful ultraviolet (UV) rays, reducing the risk of skin cancer, premature aging, and other sun-related issues. Here are some essential tips on how to carry out sun safety:

1. Use Sunscreen:

• Choose Broad-Spectrum Sunscreen: Select a sunscreen that provides broad-spectrum protection, covering both UVA and UVB rays.

• SPF 30 or Higher: Use a sunscreen with a sun protection factor (SPF) of 30 or higher for adequate protection.

• Apply Generously: Apply sunscreen generously to all exposed skin, including face, neck, ears, and any uncovered areas.

2. Reapply Sunscreen:

• Frequent Reapplication: Reapply sunscreen every two hours, or more often if swimming or sweating.

• After Swimming or Toweling Off: Reapply sunscreen after swimming or any activity that causes sweating or towel drying.

3. Wear Protective Clothing:

• Cover Exposed Skin: Wear lightweight, long-sleeved clothing to cover exposed areas.

• Choose Dark Colors: Dark-colored clothing provides more protection than light-colored fabrics.

• Use Wide-Brimmed Hats: Wear hats with wide brims to shade your face, neck, and ears.

4. Seek Shade:

• Limit Sun Exposure: Avoid prolonged sun exposure, especially during peak hours (10 a.m. to 4 p.m.).

• Use Shade Structures: Seek shade under trees, umbrellas, or other shade structures when outdoors.

5. Wear Sunglasses:

• UV-Protective Sunglasses: Choose sunglasses that provide 100% UV protection to shield your eyes from harmful rays.

• Wraparound Styles: Opt for sunglasses with wraparound styles for additional protection from the sides.

6. Plan Outdoor Activities Wisely:

• Timing Matters: Plan outdoor activities earlier in the morning or later in the afternoon to avoid the peak sun hours.

• Check UV Index: Be aware of the UV index, and plan activities accordingly. Higher UV index levels indicate stronger UV rays.

7. Stay Hydrated:

• Drink Plenty of Water: Staying hydrated is essential, especially in hot and sunny conditions.

• Limit Alcohol and Caffeine: Reduce consumption of alcohol and caffeinated beverages, as they can contribute to dehydration.

8. Be Sun Smart Near Water, Snow, and Sand:

• Reflective Surfaces: Water, snow, and sand can reflect and amplify UV rays. Take extra precautions in these environments.

• Use Extra Protection: Apply sunscreen more frequently and take additional measures to protect your skin.

9. Check Your Medications:

• Photosensitive Medications: Some medications can increase sensitivity to sunlight. Check with your healthcare provider if you're taking any photosensitive medications.

10. Practice Sun Safety for Children:

• Use Sunscreen for Kids: Choose sunscreen specifically designed for children with at least SPF 30.

• Protective Clothing: Dress children in protective clothing and hats, and keep them in shaded areas.

11. Perform Skin Self-Exams:

• Regular Skin Checks: Monitor your skin for any changes, including new moles, changes in size, shape, or color.

• Seek Professional Examination: If you notice any suspicious changes, consult a dermatologist promptly.

12. Know the ABCDEs of Melanoma:

• Asymmetry: One half of the mole does not match the other half.

• Border Irregularity: The edges are irregular, notched, or blurred.

• Color Changes: The color is not uniform and may include different shades of brown or black.

• Diameter: Melanomas are often larger than 6 millimeters in diameter.

• Evolution: Changes in size, shape, color, or elevation over time.

13. Be Mindful of Reflections:

• Car Windows and Mirrors: UV rays can penetrate car windows. Consider applying sunscreen or wearing protective clothing during extended car rides.

14. Use Sunless Tanning Products:

• Sunless Tanners: Consider using sunless tanning products if you want a tan without exposing your skin to harmful UV rays.

• Apply Evenly: Follow product instructions carefully, and apply evenly for a natural-looking tan.

15. Regular Skin Checkups:

• Dermatologist Visits: Schedule regular checkups with a dermatologist for skin examinations, especially if you have a history of skin cancer.

16. Be Sun Safe Year-Round:

• All Seasons: Practice sun safety throughout the year, not just during the summer months.

• Winter Sun Protection: Snow can reflect UV rays, so sun protection is important during winter activities.

By incorporating these sun safety practices into your routine, you can enjoy outdoor activities while minimizing the risks associated with prolonged sun exposure. Protecting your skin from harmful UV rays

Clean and safe living spaces play a crucial role in promoting overall well-being and contributing to a healthy lifestyle. Maintaining a clean and safe environment has various physical, mental, and social benefits. Here's an overview of the importance of clean and safe living spaces:

Physical Health:

• Prevention of Illness: Regular cleaning helps eliminate dust, allergens, and pathogens that can contribute to respiratory issues and allergies. A clean environment reduces the risk of infectious diseases by minimizing the presence of harmful bacteria and viruses.

• Reduced Exposure to Toxins: Proper cleaning practices limit exposure to harmful substances, such as mold, mildew, and chemical pollutants, which can impact respiratory and overall health.

• Promotion of Hygiene: Clean living spaces support personal hygiene practices, preventing the spread of germs and reducing the likelihood of infections.

• Safe Food Preparation: Clean kitchens and food preparation areas help prevent contamination, ensuring the safety of the food consumed and reducing the risk of foodborne illnesses.

Mental and Emotional Well-Being:

Stress Reduction: A clutter-free and organized living space can contribute to lower stress levels and a sense of order and control. Living in a clean environment fosters a positive mindset and reduces feelings of overwhelm.

• Improved Focus and Productivity: A clean and organized workspace enhances concentration and productivity by reducing distractions and creating a conducive atmosphere for work or study.

• Enhanced Mental Clarity: A tidy and well-maintained environment can positively impact mental clarity, making it easier to think, plan, and make decisions.

• Positive Impact on Mood: A clean and aesthetically pleasing living space can uplift mood and contribute to a more positive and optimistic outlook on life.

Social and Environmental Benefits:

• Safe Social Spaces: Clean and safe common areas, such as parks, recreational spaces, and public facilities, contribute to a sense of community and encourage social interactions.

• Community Well-Being: Maintaining cleanliness in shared spaces promotes community health and well-being, fostering a sense of pride and responsibility among residents.

• Environmental Sustainability: Adopting eco-friendly cleaning practices and waste management contributes to environmental sustainability, reducing the impact on ecosystems and natural resources.

Long-Term Health and Safety:

• Prevention of Hazards: Regular maintenance and cleaning help identify and address potential hazards, such as faulty wiring, leaks, or structural issues, ensuring a safe living environment.

• Home Safety: Clean and well-maintained homes reduce the risk of accidents and injuries, providing a safe and secure space for residents.

• Early Detection of Issues: Regular cleaning allows for the early detection of problems like water damage or pest infestations, preventing these issues from escalating into larger and more costly problems.

Quality of Sleep:

• Comfortable Sleeping Environment: Clean and well-organized bedrooms with comfortable bedding contribute to a restful sleep environment, positively impacting overall health and daily functioning.

• Reduced Allergens: Regular cleaning helps reduce allergens, dust mites, and other potential irritants, creating a healthier atmosphere for quality sleep.

Pride and Satisfaction:

• Sense of Accomplishment: Maintaining a clean living space provides a sense of accomplishment and pride, contributing to overall life satisfaction.

• Positive Lifestyle Habits: Cultivating a habit of cleanliness encourages a proactive and responsible approach to daily life, promoting positive lifestyle habits.

In summary, clean and safe living spaces are essential for maintaining good health, supporting mental well-being, fostering positive social connections, and ensuring long-term safety and sustainability. Regular cleaning, organization, and attention to environmental factors contribute to a harmonious and thriving living environment.

CONCLUSION

In conclusion, embracing a lifestyle focused on healthy living is a holistic and empowering journey that encompasses physical, mental, and social well-being. From maintaining a balanced diet and engaging in regular physical activity to fostering positive relationships and creating safe living environments, the principles of healthy living contribute to a fulfilling and vibrant life.

Prioritizing health involves not only the avoidance of harmful substances and the adoption of positive habits but also a commitment to continuous learning, self-improvement, and resilience in the face of life's challenges. Recognizing the interconnectedness of various aspects of well-being, from proper nutrition and exercise to adequate sleep and stress management, underscores the importance of a comprehensive approach to health.

By incorporating healthy practices into daily routines, individuals can experience increased vitality, mental clarity, and emotional resilience. The benefits extend beyond personal well-being, impacting the broader community through the promotion of a culture of health and well-being.

In essence, healthy living is not a destination but a continuous journey, marked by conscious choices, self-awareness, and a commitment to lifelong well-being. It is a journey that celebrates the remarkable synergy between physical health, mental resilience, and the quality of relationships, ultimately leading to a more fulfilling and purposeful existence. As we navigate this journey, let us embrace the empowering notion that our choices today profoundly shape the vitality and quality of life we experience tomorrow.

www.ingramcontent.com/pod-product-compliance
Lightning Source LLC
Chambersburg PA
CBHW050817260726

48660CB00004B/1472